Reflections on Long-Term Relational Psychotherapy and Psychoanalysis

Reflections on Long-Term Relational Psychotherapy and Psychoanalysis explores how relational analysts think about and pursue long-term therapeutic relationships in their practices. Many therapists work intensively with their clients over many years and don't necessarily talk about their work. More exploration is needed into what is taking place inside of these long-term relationships.

The chapters cover a range of topics that focus on aspects of the therapeutic relationship that are unique to long-term psychoanalytic work. They include work with various issues such as trauma, death and dying, cross-cultural issues, suffering, mourning, neuropsychoanalysis, unique endings, attachment, intimacy, and the many ways in which therapists change along with their clients as they go through life stages together.

Reflections on Long-Term Relational Psychotherapy and Psychoanalysis will be of great interest to psychoanalysts, psychodynamic psychotherapists, psychologists, social workers, workers in other mental health fields, graduate students, and anyone who is interested in change processes.

Susan A. Lord, PhD, is a Clinical Associate Professor in the Social Work Department at the University of New Hampshire, Durham, NH, USA. She is a Taos Institute Associate, an Associate Editor of the *Journal of Family Therapy,* and maintains a private practice in York, Maine.

"Susan Lord has done it again – this time pulling together a riveting collection of intimate 'stories from inside long-term treatment' written by a wide-ranging group of gifted 'relational' clinicians: a group that is diversified with respect to training and orientation but that shares a common bond, namely, a passion for cutting deep and broad; infinite compassion and heart; tremendous courage and determination; strong belief in the transformative power of 'mutuality' and 'relationship'; keen ability to negotiate therapeutic impasses; indestructibility and capacity to survive relational turbulence; and unwavering faith in the psychotherapeutic process as a means of effecting enduring and characterological change. Lord, who clearly holds 'moments of authentic meeting' as central to the work of healing old wounds and facilitating the emergence of new possibilities, is offering readers (whatever their level of expertise or therapeutic approach) the rare opportunity of peeking into the sacrosanct chambers of experienced clinicians who are daring to reveal tender, loving, and vulnerable details about how they enable clients to triumph over their internal demons and realize their potential. In response to the frequently asked question, 'How long will this take?' I have often found myself responding, 'It depends upon how ambitious we are.' The beautifully and compellingly crafted narratives in this generous and tender volume certainly speak to the reality that if client and therapist dare to dream big and aim high, then the sky is truly the limit; the vignettes reinforce the idea that 'you should shoot for the moon because, if you miss, you'll still land among the stars.' Bravo to the thirteen therapists who first gave their hearts to their clients and are now giving their hearts to us. Thank you, Dr. Lord."

– **Martha Stark, MD,** Faculty, Harvard Medical School; Co-Founder/Co-Director/ Faculty, Center for Psychoanalytic Studies; award-winning author of 7 books including *Relentless Hope: The Refusal to Grieve*

"This edited collection makes an important contribution to the literature on longer-term analytic treatments. Susan Lord has invited an interesting group of authors who grapple with the knotty question of 'How long is "enough" treatment?' These authors make the solid case that developmental relational traumas leave deep lasting internal injuries that may require longer-term treatments. Threaded through the chapters are case examples demonstrating the hallmarks of effective relational treatment: empathy, recognition, authenticity, attunement and the complexities of attachment ruptures and repair within the context of trauma histories. This book should become required reading for those in mental health training and for practitioners in the field."

– **Jill Salberg, PhD, ABPP,** Clinical Associate Professor and Clinical Consultant/Supervisor, New York University Postdoctoral Program in Psychotherapy and Psychoanalysis; Faculty and Supervisor, The Stephen Mitchell Center for Relational Studies, The Institute for Contemporary Psychotherapy; Visiting Faculty, Tel Aviv University, School of Continuing Medical Education; Editor, *Good Enough Endings: Breaks, Interruptions and Terminations from Contemporary Relational Perspectives* (2010)

"Concepts of time and the illusion of timelessness are central to understanding both the unconscious and psychoanalysis. Still, few if any books address these notions as they directly impact treatment duration. Susan Lord's excellent collection is a welcome exception. She and an outstanding roster of contemporary contributors turn a relational lens to questions as old as psychoanalysis itself: How much is enough? Is there such a thing as too long? This book belongs on the shelf of anyone who is interested in the study and practice of psychoanalysis."

– **Steven Kuchuck, DSW,** President, International Association of Relational Psychoanalysis and Psychotherapy; Editor, *Clinical Implications of the Psychoanalyst's Life Experience: When the Personal Becomes Professional*

Reflections on Long-Term Relational Psychotherapy and Psychoanalysis

Relational Analysis Interminable

Edited by Susan A. Lord

Routledge
Taylor & Francis Group
LONDON AND NEW YORK

First published 2019
by Routledge
2 Park Square, Milton Park, Abingdon, Oxon OX14 4RN

and by Routledge
52 Vanderbilt Avenue, New York, NY 10017

Routledge is an imprint of the Taylor & Francis Group, an informa business

British Library Cataloguing in Publication Data
A catalogue record for this book is available from the British Library

Library of Congress Cataloging in Publication Data
Names: Lord, Susan (Susan A.), editor.
Title: Reflections on long-term relational psychotherapy and psychoanalysis: relational analysis interminable/edited by Susan A. Lord.
Description: Abingdon, Oxon; New York, NY: Routledge, 2019. | Includes bibliographical references and index.
Identifiers: LCCN 2018050749 (print) | LCCN 2018052122 (ebook) | ISBN 9780429054501 (Master) | ISBN 9780429620256 (ePub) | ISBN 9780429618109 (MobiPocket) | ISBN 9780429622403 (Web Pdf) | ISBN 9780367150150 (hardback: alk. paper) | ISBN 9780367150167 (pbk.: alk. paper) | ISBN 9780429054501 (ebk)
Subjects: | MESH: Psychotherapy–methods | Psychoanalytic Therapy–methods | Professional-Patient Relations
Classification: LCC RC480.5 (ebook) | LCC RC480.5 (print) | NLM WM 420 | DDC 616.89/14–dc23
LC r

ISBN: 978-0-367-15015-0 (hbk)
ISBN: 978-0-367-15016-7 (pbk)
ISBN: 978-0-429-05450-1 (ebk)

Typeset in Times New Roman
by Swales & Willis, Exeter, Devon, UK

For
Sarah Currier Holbrook

Contents

List of contributors ix
Acknowledgments xii
Introduction xiii

PART I
The terrain **1**

1 An interview with Joyce Edward 3
JOYCE EDWARD AND SUSAN LORD

2 Long-term psychotherapy: Whyever not? (A question of assumptions) 9
PATRICIA DEYOUNG

3 It takes as long as it takes: Therapists' subjective experiences of long-term therapy 27
JEAN KOTCHER

4 In defense of long-term treatment: On the vanishing holding environment 37
WILLIAM S. MEYER

5 Long-term treatment in the rearview mirror 50
WILLIAM S. MEYER

PART II
Trauma and issues of attachment **59**

6 Mourning the melancholy object: Giving voice to traumatic experience 61
CAROL GANZER

7 The role of ethnicity and culture in the long-term treatment of childhood trauma 74
SHOSHANA RINGEL

8 It takes a long time to grow young: Working relationally with developmental trauma 86
NATALIE PEACOCK-CORRAL

9 Masks, walls and metaphors: Reflections on long-term treatment 101
KATHLEEN FARGIONE

PART III
How could it be otherwise? 117

10 Being still: Sitting with suffering in long-term relational practice 119
JOAN BERZOFF

11 Till death do us part: Relational work and terminal illness 132
SUSAN LORD

12 Looking back through 38 years of practicing relational psychoanalysis in search of answers to the question of interminability 141
STEFANIE SOLOW GLENNON

13 Neuropsychoanalysis and the repressed: Rendering what is possible in long-term psychotherapy 152
JANE ABRAMS

14 The longest goodbyes: Analysis everlasting 166
ANTHONY BASS

Index 183

Contributors

Jane Abrams, DSW, LCSW, is a lecturer in the MSW program and on the faculty of the DSW program at the School of Social Policy and Practice at the University of Pennsylvania. She is an alumnus of the Psychoanalytic and Psychodynamic Teachers' Academy of the American Psychoanalytic Association and is on the faculty of the newly established Undergraduate Minor in Psychoanalytic Studies at the University of Pennsylvania. She maintains a private practice in Philadelphia, specializing in treating adult survivors of childhood trauma, couples therapy, and clinical supervision.

Anthony Bass, PhD, is on the faculty and is a supervising analyst at the New York University Postdoctoral Program in Psychoanalysis and Psychotherapy. He is also on the teaching and supervisory faculty of many training programs and institutes around the country, including the Relational Psychoanalysis of Philadelphia, the National Institute for the Psychotherapies National Training Program, and the Stephen A. Mitchell Center for Relational Studies in New York City, for which he serves as president. He is the joint editor in chief of *Psychoanalytic Dialogues, The International Journal of Relational Perspectives*, and a founding and current director of the International Association for Relational Psychoanalysis and Psychotherapy. His practice in New York City includes psychoanalysis, psychotherapy, couples and family therapy, and supervisory consultation.

Joan Berzoff, EdD, is Professor Emerita, Smith College School for Social Work. She is the author of several books, including *Inside Out and Outside In, Falling through the Cracks*, and *Living with Dying*. She maintains a private practice in Northampton, MA.

Patricia DeYoung, MSW, PhD, is a founding faculty member of the Toronto Institute for Relational Psychotherapy. Her books include *Relational Psychotherapy: A Primer*, and *Understanding and Treating Chronic Shame: A Relational/Neurobiological Approach*. She maintains a private clinical and supervisory practice in Toronto, specializing in relational modes of individual and couples therapy.

Joyce Edward, MSSA, is a 94-year-old retired psychoanalytic social worker who began her career in 1947. She was in private practice from 1972 until her retirement, and was an instructor at Adelphi University, Hunter College School of Social Work and Smith College School of Social Work. She authored a number of books, including *Separation/Individuation, The Sibling Relationship*, and *The Social Work Psychoanalyst's Casebook*.

Kathleen Fargione, LICSW, is a professor at the University of St. Thomas's graduate school of Social Work and at the Minnesota Psychoanalytic Society and Institute. She is a member of the American Association of Psychoanalysis and Clinical Social Work, Chapter 39 of the American Psychological Association, and the Minnesota Society for Clinical Social Workers. Her paper "Climbing a Waterfall: Understanding an Adolescent Boy in Autistic Retreat" was published in the British *Journal of Child Psychotherapy* in 2013. She is an adolescent and adult psychotherapist in Minneapolis, MN.

Carol Ganzer, PhD, is President and faculty at the Chicago Center for Psychoanalysis. She is on the faculty at the Institute for Clinical Social Work, a Lecturer at the University of Chicago, School of Social Service Administration, and instructor in the Professional Development Program's Advanced Psychodynamic Fellowship in Clinical Practice. She serves as Managing Editor of *Clinical Social Work Journal* and was previously on the Editorial Board. She is in private practice of psychoanalysis, psychotherapy, and consultation in Chicago.

Stefanie Solow Glennon, PhD, is supervising analyst at the NYU Postdoctoral Program in Psychotherapy and Psychoanalysis, teaching faculty, Stephen Mitchell Center for Relational Studies in NYC and teaching faculty, supervising analyst, member of the Training Committee at the Institute for Contemporary Psychotherapy in NYC. Dr. Glennon sits on the Editorial Board of *Psychoanalytic Dialogues*, and has written in the areas of immediate experience, obesity, mourning, artistic expression, termination, solitude, therapeutic action, and neuroscience and psychoanalysis. She is in private practice in NYC.

Jean Kotcher, PhD, is academic consulting faculty at The Sanville Institute in Berkeley, CA. In 2016, she published a book review for the *Journal of Psychoanalytic Social Work* on Judith Kantrowitz's, *Myths of Termination: What Patients Can Teach Psychoanalysts about Endings.* Dr. Kotcher conducted a study and has written on the therapist's experience of long-term therapy. She is in private practice in San Francisco, CA.

Susan Lord, PhD, LICSW, is a Clinical Associate Professor in the Social Work Department at the University of New Hampshire, Durham, NH. She is the author of the books *Moments of Meeting in Psychoanalysis* and *Wealth and Social Responsibility*, and of several book chapters and articles on work with complex childhood trauma and the use of mindfulness practices in psychotherapy. She is an Associate Editor of the *Journal of Family Therapy*, a Taos Institute Associate, and is in private practice in York, ME.

William S. Meyer, MSW, is Director of Training for the Department of Social Work and an Associate Professor in the Departments of Psychiatry and Ob/Gyn at Duke University Medical Center. He is on the faculty of the Psychoanalytic Education Center of the Carolinas and holds faculty appointments at The University of North Carolina and Smith College. He has lectured and written extensively on mental health-related topics. He is in private practice in Durham, North Carolina.

Natalie Peacock-Corral, MSW, is a graduate of the Psychoanalytic Education Center of the Carolinas Advanced Psychotherapy Training Program and is on their teaching faculty. She is the director and regular discussant of the Mindplay Program for Playmakers Theatre and the North Carolina Psychoanalytic Society in Chapel Hill, NC. She is currently in private practice in Raleigh, North Carolina.

Shoshana Ringel, PhD, is an Associate Professor at the University of Maryland School of Social Work, and is also a psychoanalyst in private practice in Baltimore, MD. She has published numerous clinical papers and co-authored three books on attachment, relational social work, and trauma. She is in private practice in Baltimore, MD.

Acknowledgments

I am forever grateful that I have the privilege of doing this work. I am blessed to be surrounded by family, friends and colleagues who support me and enliven my inner and outer worlds every day.

Thank you to Paul Russell, who taught me that relationship and risk-taking are the keys to a well-lived life.

I am lucky to have wonderful UNH and Taos Institute colleagues whose wisdom, friendship and support have encouraged me in my work. Thank you to dear friends Maryann Plunkett, Jay O. Sanders, Duncan Adams and Robert Cummins. And to my family, whose love and belief in me hold me and help to make this work possible: Ray and Priscilla Lord, Nancy Fascione, Sarah Holbrook, Andy Lord, and especially to Karen Frarie, Tessa Smith and Aleksa Smith.

Thank you to Publisher Kate Hawes and Editorial Assistant Charles Bath at Routledge who expertly guided me through and supported this project. And to all of the authors who so generously contributed their hearts and their minds to the book.

Most importantly, thank you to my clients, supervisees and students who have been such an inspiration and have helped me to grow in so many ways throughout my career.

Introduction

Susan Lord

Oliver Sacks spoke of his more-than-47-year analysis with Leonard Shengold in a 2011 interview:

> No doubt this is one of the longest analyses on record, or at least I like to think so ... *I think also we're beginning to get somewhere now* (emphasis mine). But Shengold and I have grown old together and have gone through life stages together. I still think of him as Dr. Shengold. I don't even think of his first name, and I'm always Dr. Sacks to him. The propriety is always there, but it is because the proprieties are there that there can be such freedom of communication.
>
> (Sacks, 2011)

That statement, "we're beginning to get somewhere now" is one that speaks to the crux of the matter for me. How can we know where we are going in an analysis, and how do we discern whether and when we have gotten somewhere? Does having an end in sight facilitate the process, as many have theorized? Or does it merely organize us in ways that may interfere with or promote relationship and growth? Punctuation changes things, but how?

From its inception, analysis has struggled with the question of how to structure this most real and most unreal relationship that human beings are able to pursue (Ferenczi, 1955 [1927]; Ferenczi & Rank, 1924; Freud, 1937; Rank, 1993 [1924]). In "Analysis Terminable and Interminable" Freud wrote:

> Experience has taught us that psycho-analytic therapy – the liberation of a human being from his neurotic symptoms, inhibitions and abnormalities of character – is a lengthy business. Hence, from the very beginning, attempts have been made to shorten the course of analysis.
>
> (1937, p. 211)

With the evolution of relational analysis[1] the question of when to end the analytic relationship has become even more complex. For in relational work the relationship becomes intensely real, intersubjective, collaborative, and we do go through life stages together over time as we affect and are affected by each another. As Glennon has said, "few people would willingly terminate an intense relationship that is loving, supportive, mutual, and meaningful even if more therapeutic work is not deemed necessary" (2010, p. 257). And Davies, "the significant emotional engagement and participation of the relational analyst could, in the end, leave particular patients extremely vulnerable to an experience of having been seduced and then abandoned" (2005, p. 784). Mitchell observed that there is "less useful literature on the termination of analysis than on any other major feature of the work" (1997, p. 26).

This book brings together an array of analysts and psychotherapists to grapple with the topic of long-term treatment and to offer case studies of long-term treatment relationships that they have participated in. In the development of this book I have asked the authors to answer the following questions: How do you define long-term treatment? What is the longest period of time that you have worked with a client? Is there such a thing as "analysis interminable"? How do you decide when to terminate with a client? How do you conceptualize longer-term treatment relationships? Might an analysis continue until the death or inability of one of the participants to go on?

This is a particularly poignant topic for me, as I never had the opportunity to experience a proper ending to my own treatment relationship. My analyst died precipitously of pancreatic cancer in the fifteenth year of our work together. I vividly remember his wife calling me one day during his August "vacation" to tell me that he was ill and would not be returning to his practice. I saw him one more time – in October of that year. He was greatly diminished, having lost probably half of his body weight. I could still find him in his eyes, though; his heart shone there. I told him that I would be fine. We had done the work that we needed to do. I had continued to see him because I loved him, and I had always known that one of us would have to die for our relationship to end. He left the world too soon, and we did not have time for a formal termination.

And so, I come to this book honestly, with questions: How long is too long? How long is "enough"? These are important questions for any analyst and patient to consider as they enter into this most important and, I believe, sacred relationship. Ironically though, these are questions that cannot be answered without having entered into the experience and container of a long-term therapeutic relationship.

Long-term work is something that I do. I often joke that my definition of brief treatment is anything less than 20 years. I have found that many people in our profession engage in long-term treatment relationships and don't necessarily talk about them or have a frame for them. In some ways it seems that we carry a shameful secret. Is it unethical? Unprofessional? Verboten?

In the current climate of "managed care" and briefer treatments, I am intrigued to discover what is happening within the sanctuary of our practices. What are we offering to our clients? What do we believe is possible? Each of the following chapters includes relevant theoretical material, case examples, and some discussion about the authors' views of and experiences with long-term treatment in their practices.

The book is divided into three sections: "The Terrain", "Trauma and Issues of Attachment", and "How Could it Be Otherwise?" We begin with an interview with Joyce Edwards, a 94-year-old analyst who had been in practice for 60 years before she retired at the age of 83. She offers her long-range view of long-term treatment and discusses some of the issues she sees as particularly important as they have evolved over time. In Chapter 2 Patricia DeYoung offers the compelling view that we should leave the decisions about length of treatment to our clients. She questions our assumptions about long-term treatment and goes on to discuss the many complicated factors that go into decisions about length of treatment and the relationships that follow.

Chapter 3, by Jean Kotcher, offers the results of a study she performed in 2012, in which she interviewed therapists to learn about their views of and experiences with long-term treatment. In Chapter 4, a reprint of a classic article written by William Meyer in 1993, we revisit his compelling arguments for sustaining the holding environments that he believes our clients need and deserve, and learn that things have not changed much, as the current terrain is remarkably similar to that of 25 years ago. Meyer offers an update on these issues in Chapter 5 and fills us in on what has happened in his work with the client, Sue, that he discussed in that article. He beautifully and movingly describes how their long-term and sometimes unorthodox relationship sustained and enriched both of their lives over the years.

Part II, "Trauma and Issues of Attachment" begins with Carol Ganzer's chapter on mourning the melancholy object. Through an object relations lens, she explores issues of loss and grief, focusing on the "present absence(s)" that can invade current relationships. Shosana Ringel, in Chapter 7, writes about cultural issues in a non-traditional long-term treatment relationship with an Asian client who had a trauma history, and the healing work that they were able to do together that was perhaps enhanced by the fact that they were both immigrants from different cultures.

Natalie Peacock-Corral writes in Chapter 8 about her growth and development as a young and inexperienced clinician working with a challenging client through two pregnancies and a miscarriage, finally using music as a breakthrough way of communicating, connccting and moving forward. In Chapter 9 Fargione focuses in on the importance of long-term treatment to rebuild missing pieces in psychic structures, repairing "internalized and damaged objects"; she emphasizes that this difficult and often painful work takes time.

Part III opens with Joan Berzoff's chapter addressing the importance of sitting with and bearing witness to suffering. She offers several cases studies as illustrations and points out the paradox that sitting with suffering may offer hope and improve our capacities to bear the suffering that is, to varying degrees, an inevitable part of every human life. In Chapter 11, I write about a 25-year therapy relationship that is ending as my client is dying of stage 4 cancer. I talk about my countertransference responses, the mutual growth that we have shared over the years of working together, and the intimate knowing that has evolved. Stefanie Solow Glennon's Chapter 12 reflects on her 38 years of practicing relational psychoanalysis. She explores the question of whether some analyses should be interminable and, if so, which ones need to be interminable.

In Chapter 13 Jane Abrams introduces concepts from neuropsychoanalysis, discussing the brain's capacities to remember, and the importance of adaptation and hopefulness in getting our needs met. She talks about how experience in a safe and holding relationship can change the brain. In the final chapter Anthony Bass looks back over his long career, exploring some of the characteristics of long-term work and the reality that each analysis is unique, and we can't know what the terrain will be or what the relationship will bring.

> Each patient's (and analyst's) sense of what might be a desirable and achievable goal of analysis over time will inevitably change along the way, as awareness expands, perspectives shift, and the patient comes to see emergent aspects of what brought her to analysis in the first place, and what might constitute an acceptable endpoint.

This book begins with many questions about long-term treatment, and with a discussion about assumptions that we may make as we enter into the mutuality of long-term therapeutic relationships. In the end it seems that there are many views and practices, as there are many practitioners and patients. I am not interested in reaching any conclusions here, but rather in opening and promoting ongoing conversations as theories and practices evolve. It is my hope that there will continue to be multiple points of departure for the interminable exploration of the deeply satisfying and sustaining mutual relationships that can be developed in long-term psychoanalytic work.

Note

1 The terms psychoanalyst and psychotherapist are used interchangeably throughout the book to signify clinicians who identify with psychoanalytic ideas and practices.

References

Davies, J. M. (2005). Transformations of desire and despair: Reflections on the termination process. *Psychoanalytic Dialogues, 15*(6), 779–805.

Ferenczi, S. (1955 [1927]). The problem of termination of the analysis. In M. Balint (Ed.), *Final contributions to the problems and methods of psychoanalysis* (pp. 77–86). London: Hogarth.

Ferenczi, S. & Rank, O. (1924). *The development of psychoanalysis.* New York, NY & Washington, DC: *Nervous and Mental Disease Monograph Series* (No. 40).

Freud, S. (1937). Analysis terminable and interminable. In J. Strachey (Ed.), *The standard edition of the complete works of Sigmund Freud* (Vol. 23, pp. 211–253). London: Hogarth.

Glennon, S. S. (2010). Relational analyses: Are they more difficult to terminate? In J. Salberg (Ed.), *Good enough endings* (pp. 257–275). New York, NY: Routledge.

Mitchell, S. A. (1997). *Influence and autonomy in psychoanalysis.* Hillsdale, NJ: Analytic Press.

Rank, O. (1993 [1924]). *The trauma of birth.* New York, NY: Dover Publishing.

Sacks, O. (2011). "The longest running psychoanalysis on record." Retrieved from www.webofstories.com/play/oliver.sacks/196.

Salberg, J. (Ed.). (2010). *Good enough endings: Breaks, interruptions and terminations from contemporary relational perspectives.* New York, NY: Routledge.

Part I

The terrain

Chapter 1

An interview with Joyce Edward

Joyce Edward and Susan Lord

As I was putting together this book it became clear to me that it would be important to include voices of senior psychotherapists and analysts in order to gain their long-range perspectives on long-term treatment. This chapter offers an interview with Joyce Edward, a 94-year-old psychodynamic social worker and analyst whose career began in 1947 and continued until her retirement in 2007, a total of 60 years. As a clinician who trained with such esteemed analysts as Gertrude and Ruben Blanck, Margaret Mahler, Martin Bergman, Lawrence Friedman, Jacob Arlow and Roy Schafer, Joyce offers a particular view on the evolution of long-term relational psychoanalysis.

Joyce earned her MSSA from Case Western Reserve University in 1946. She began her career at Central Islip State Hospital in 1947, moving to the Nassau County Department of Welfare Children's Services in 1948. From 1956 to 1969 she worked as a caseworker and supervised clinicians and teachers working with emotionally disturbed children at a therapeutic school. She trained in psychoanalysis and psychotherapy at the Institute for the Study of Psychotherapy in New York, and maintained a private practice from 1972 until her retirement in 2007. Joyce was an instructor at Adelphi University, Hunter College School of Social Work and Smith College School of Social Work for more than 20 years, and also taught at the Society for Psychoanalytic Study and Research and the New York School for Psychoanalytic Psychotherapy.

Joyce is the author of many articles and books on aspects of psychotherapy and psychoanalysis. She wrote *The Sibling Relationship: A Force for Growth and Conflict* (2010), co-authored *Separation-Individuation: Theory and Application* (1991), and co-edited *Fostering Healing and Growth: A Psychoanalytic Social Work Approach* (1996) and *The Social Work Psychoanalyst's Casebook: Clinical Voices in Honor of Jean Sanville* (1999). Known for her advocacy work on behalf of clients' rights, particularly in the area of confidentiality and access to services, Joyce was co-founder and first co-chair of the National Coalition for Mental Health Professionals and Consumers in New York.

Joyce has some very strong ideas about the ways in which managed care interferes with long-term work, and her coalition work was a part of her pursuit of social justice in this regard. Here is an excerpt from Joyce's writing about managed care and its impact on psychodynamic work:

> Managed mental health care is not psychotherapy. Instead it is what it says it is, an arrangement designed to *manage* people, both patients and therapists. Whereas for the psychotherapist, self-determination is both a means and a goal of treatment, corporate mental health care places serious limits on the freedom of both patients and therapists to determine the means and goals of their work together. The restriction of freedom is perhaps one of the most deleterious characteristics of the managed care system. In depriving individuals of their privacy and of the assurance that their confidentiality can be protected, patients are being deprived of the freedom to speak openly, thereby compromising one of the most basic constituents of the therapeutic process. At the same time, the limited numbers of sessions being offered, and the sudden changes in therapists that are occasioned by companies merging or closing or by the unexplained termination of therapists from panels, are impeding the establishment of a sound therapeutic relationship, the second major constituent of sound psychodynamically-oriented treatment. When these two major constituents of treatment, a free and open communicative process and the establishment of a therapeutic relationship are absent, is psychodynamic therapy possible?
>
> (1998, p. 114)

That final question is an important one that I believe speaks to the central issue. Communication and relationship are core elements of the therapeutic endeavor and must be developed freely without the constraints of time limits or other external regulations. Long-term work certainly offers the opportunity to freely develop both and, with the advent of relational work, it has become even more critical that there is an opportunity for interactions to evolve without constraint.

Joyce is highly regarded for her writing, her teaching, her curiosity and openness and her consummate generosity of spirit. This interview took place in her home in Long Island, New York, where she graciously served me a wonderful lunch and shared her wisdom and her views on long-term treatment. As I sat with her I was able to experience her warmth, her humor, and her passion for social justice in the interview that follows.

Definitions

Susan: Thank you so much for agreeing to talk with me. I am interested in your views on long-term treatment. First, how would you define long-term treatment?

Joyce: While I was in practice I probably thought of long-term treatment as treatment that would go beyond six or seven years. In my own practice three to five years seemed to be the average length of time I saw a patient. It is important to note that in those days psychotherapy patients were frequently seen by therapists like myself twice a week, and psychoanalytic patients three or four times a week. Fees were often reduced in order to provide patients with what we saw as more favorable treatment arrangements. Several of my colleagues were in analysis for more than 20 years. I know two women who have been in treatment on and off for most of their lives, to what they regard as their great benefit.

Susan: What was the longest period of time that you worked with a client?

Joyce: Over the years I have actually only treated one person in what I considered to be long-term treatment. I probably saw him for about 13 years. After about five years of my work with him I became concerned about the limited gains he was making and sought a consultation. What was I missing? Might I be doing something to hold on to the patient? I was surprised when the consultant, reminding me that the patient had been in one treatment or another since adolescence, referred to the patient as a "lifer." He saw the patient's need for lifelong treatment as related to the severe traumas the patient had experienced early in life, and the absence of any significant support figure in his life. He pointed to the few but significant gains the patient had made through our work together and emphasized the importance of the therapeutic relationship in fostering the patient's continued stability.

In retrospect I realize that what we needed to explore in that consultation was my discomfort with the idea of lifelong treatments. What was it stirring up in me? Like some other analysts of my times I was suspicious of long-term treatments. Were they not the result of therapists holding on to their patients for their own gain either psychologically or financially, or both?

Our work together was brought to a close by my retirement. At that point the patient felt he was much stronger, and decided he would like to see how he would fare without treatment. However, I learned from the therapist, whose name I had given him should he wish to continue with someone else, that within the year he had begun a new treatment. While my colleague has been appropriately protective of the patient's privacy and confidentiality, she has shared the fact that the patient has done well over the intervening years, and was being seen on a once-a-month basis at the time I spoke with her.

When I look back on this case, I see how right the consultant was. The patient was a "lifer" and what I ask now is "what is wrong with that?" In retrospect, why might a man who had suffered the loss of both parents during his first two years and then faced ever-changing caretakers for the rest of his childhood, not seek a supportive therapist for the years to come?

Brief treatment

Susan: When you were trained were you trained to do briefer work?

Joyce: Actually no. I was trained by Gertrude and Rubin Blanck who regarded twice a week or preferably three times a week sessions as optimum arrangements. I don't recall though any consideration given to the length of time of treatment. However, students at the Blanck Institute tended to work with severely troubled patients and were prepared for their treatments to take time.

I also studied with Jacob Arlow. We were a group of social workers. I don't recall any discussion of the length of treatment. However, Dr. Arlow apparently noted some urgency in our work to help the patient sooner rather than later. He accused us of a "compulsion to cure."

There was, during that time, interest on the part of some psychoanalysts in brief treatment. I no longer recall the group that was developing what was referred to by some as "time-limited" treatment. However, I do recall a patient I saw after they had been in such a program. Discharged after the ten agreed-upon sessions, the patient had in the initial session with me noted that he had "failed" his earlier treatment.

When managed care came along, brief treatments became standard. One of the reasons therapists like myself organized the National Coalition for Mental Health Professionals and Consumers that you mentioned, was our deep concern about the limited number of sessions that companies were willing to authorize.

Analysis interminable?

Susan: What do you think about therapists and their clients continuing their work indefinitely? Until one of them dies or is unable to continue?

Joyce: I have unfortunately known therapists who have worked until they died or were unable to continue to work. I have treated two patients whose therapists were seriously ill and died during the treatment. One died during a session! The impact on both these patients was profoundly disturbing.

I also felt that the therapists suffered for continuing to work through their illnesses which, to my knowledge, they did not apprize their patients of until it was impossible to conceal. While the therapists found the work helpful to them, they were aware I think of the potential harm they might be doing to their patients, and troubled by this. Also they found it increasingly difficult to conduct the treatment in the excellent way they had before.

I have always favored retiring when one is fit and able to do so voluntarily. I stopped taking new patients in my early seventies and retired at 83. I am glad that I did so. I loved the work. It was so personally rewarding, I felt like I was being helpful and I gained great satisfaction from feeling like I was continuing to learn and develop, a bonus our profession offers us. However, I have not missed the work. I actually feel relieved not to have the responsibilities that are entailed.

Sometimes when I hear therapist friends talking about a case, I feel I could no longer deal with the challenges they are facing. I could not take the sadness that we therapists often have to "hold." Like many other elderly persons, I have had to face many losses over the years. They come more frequently as one grows older. I have several ill friends that I try to support to the best of my ability. I feel now that it would be much harder for me to listen fully to the painful material that as therapists we listen to and try to help our patients with.

Future

Susan: How do you think things will develop with long-term treatment over time?

Joyce: The future of long-term treatment is in some ways tied up with the future of psychoanalysis. At the moment, that future seems very uncertain. Woody Allen's long analysis has long been used to disparage psychoanalysis, and it is not unusual for lay persons to ascribe greed on the part of analysts to a particular person's lengthy treatment. If it is not the analyst holding on to the patient, it is the patient's "dependency" that is often said to be offensive.

I can only hope that somehow the public will in time awaken more fully to the deleterious effects of deprivation and trauma on human development and the need for a psychodynamically oriented treatment that can help ameliorate the ill effects of past noxious experiences and foster continuing development.

I do think in the end that it's all about the relationship. I hate to say that in a way, because we work so hard to learn a lot of things. I always remember a case that I had. One of my first patients had just been released from the hospital, she had made a suicide attempt. I saw her for two years and she got better and left, then she came back and did more work and left again. Years went by and she wrote me a letter. She came back to visit and to show me her two kids. She came to the front door. I sat with her and her two kids, and she said, "Would you like to know what helped me? You listened so. You seemed to think what I said was important." And I thought, all these years and interpretations ... I think bearing witness is very important too. There had been terrible abuse in this family, and it was important to have someone know and indicate that this really was awful and it shouldn't have happened. You wish you were there to stop it, but you can't.

I am hopeful that a volume such as this will help clinicians appreciate that there are some individuals for whom long-term, sometimes several intermittent treatments or continued treatment through life are the "treatments of choice." For some of these "lifers," their treatment may remain essential in the absence of supportive figures. For some, their goals for self-development will lead them to long-term treatments. For others changes along the life cycle, traumatic experiences, losses or other major events will bring them back to treatment.

While I am far more comfortable with long-term treatments than I was earlier in my career, I do believe that it is important that we carefully evaluate our work with our clients as we proceed. There are treatments that are prolonged due to a therapist's limitations. Countertransferences, lack of skills on the part of the therapist, poor fit between therapist and patient, and any other number of factors may render a treatment ineffective or even harmful to a client. The importance of self-supervision, consultations with more experienced therapists, group consultations and the highest standard of professional ethics cannot be overemphasized.

References

Edward, J. (1998). Impact of managed care on psychodynamic treatment (book). *Clinical Social Work Journal, 26*(1), 111–114.

Edward, J. (2010). *The sibling relationship: A force for growth and conflict*. Lanham, MD: Jason Aronson.

Edward, J. & Rose, E. (eds.). (1999). *The social work psychoanalyst's casebook: Clinical voices in honor of Jean Sanville*. Hillsdale, NJ: The Analytic Press.

Edward, J., Ruskin, N. & Tunini, P. (eds.). (1991). *Separation-individuation: Theory and application*, 2nd ed. New York: Gardner Press.

Edward, J. & Sanville, J. (eds.). (1996). *Fostering healing and growth: A psychoanalytic social work approach*. Northvale, NJ: Jason Aronson.

Chapter 2

Long-term psychotherapy

Whyever not? (A question of assumptions)

Patricia DeYoung

As do most relational therapists in private practice, I leave the question of "How long shall we work together?" to my clients. A few need only a brief stint of help. Many want to invest longer term in their psychological well-being, and some have the means to do so. Some can afford only what their insurance allows. Others, who have little or no coverage, continue only for as long as they feel desperate.

So that's one answer to the question, "Whyever *not* long-term?" Because it can be too expensive. For therapists who work in social service agencies and mental health centers, psychotherapy has been made a scarce resource, the number of sessions limited. Fortunately, sometimes brief work is exactly what's needed. Some clients are quickly able to identify options, work with emotions, or try new patterns; they finish brief therapy with a new sense of self-understanding and accomplishment. Here is a second answer to the question, "Whyever not long-term?" Because sometimes it isn't necessary.

But often, for other clients, it is necessary. We have all worked with clients who have suffered developmental relational trauma, who struggle with chronic anxiety, isolation, and self-loathing, and yet are able to hold themselves together well enough to work and thus pay for the therapy that helps them in a long trajectory of recovery. And then there are the people we don't see because they can't afford us, the relationally traumatized people whose psychological fragility has blocked their access to a standard of living that would allow them to pay for treatment that leads to recovery and well-being.

As a relational psychotherapist, I assume that for people in both groups a relationship with an understanding, trustworthy person is foundational to treatment. It takes time for such a relationship to develop and then to generate change. But if such long-term therapy is what relationally traumatized people need most, whyever would it be withheld? It's a matter of assumptions.

We could question the assumption that such therapy is "too expensive." Yes, the annual cost of weekly psychotherapy could be more than the annual cost of psychotropic medication. But it is not the cost of surgery in an operating theater, the cost of a series of CAT scans and MRIs, or the cost of an annual psychiatric inpatient stabilization for several weeks. The psychotherapy needed by people in chronic emotional pain need is "too expensive" because in our culture, people in disabling emotional pain aren't taken seriously – unless they threaten physical harm to self or others or they are suddenly unable to fulfill their responsibilities. Then their subjective suffering is objectified, reduced to a list of symptoms that become targets for medication. The goal is to hit the targets (albeit with side effects), so that these vulnerable folks can achieve or return to a life of "normalcy" or "productivity," able to ignore or push through their alienation, isolation, and self-loathing.

When as relational therapists we privilege our clients' subjective experiences of suffering and of well-being in relation to self and others, we are taking a stand against a large, complex system of assumptions. The argument for objective symptom relief through medication is but a small part of the system. The system is a worldview, a way of life, a web of belief; here is but a short, spare list of the assumptions it generates that shape practices around "mental health."

- The value of persons lies in their productivity, in what they do.
- Human well-being should be assessed against physical and mental measures of "normal."
- Mental disorders are the same sort of phenomena as the biophysical disorders defined by Western medicine.
- Treatment requires a specific kind of assessment: a diagnosis of mental disorder based on a compilation of symptoms.
- Diagnosis should be matched with the pharmacological and/or psychotherapeutic interventions that have been shown to be effective in treating the disorder in question.
- Studies that test for significant relationships between certain modes of treatment and the relief of symptoms provide reliable measures of the efficacy of psychotherapy as well as of psychopharmacology.

These assumptions do not in themselves create a bias toward brief treatment. In this version of reality, what matters is that treatment reduces the symptoms that comprise a disorder. And then, of course, the more cost-effective these treatments are, the better. The gold standard is disorder-specific, manualized, measurably effective intervention that is also as brief as possible.

All systems of belief and conviction are highly resistant to argument. Rather than quarrel with this one, I would like simply to present an alternative set of beliefs and assumptions:

- The value of persons lies in their subjective being, not in their doing or productivity.

- Well-being is a matter of persons' subjective experience across a wide range of typical and atypical life situations – physical, mental, psychological, and relational.
- Some symptoms of "mental disorders" are the result of biophysical disorders, but a large majority are symptoms of persons' damaged relationships with their social world.
- Treatment requires an assessment of persons' subjective experience of psychological distress in the context of their life situations; it focuses on how their distress interacts with their capacities for self-reflection, agency, and meaningful connection with others.
- To relieve emotional and psychological pain, appropriate medication may be matched with specific symptoms (no "disorder" required), but medication is given only in the context of conversation (psychotherapy) that explores the person's experiences of self and self-with-other that are painful or disturbing; this may include the experience of taking medication.
- Studies to test the efficacy of such psychotherapy would measure changes in clients' capacities for self-reflective, agentic relationship with self and with others, noting related changes in symptoms, and they would test for significant connections between these changes for the better and therapists' specific modes of working with the therapeutic relationship.

Note that these assumptions do not, in themselves, mandate long-term psychotherapy. What they support is psychotherapy that attends to a whole person within complex social contexts, and that takes whatever time is required to create a trustworthy therapeutic relationship.

"Whatever time is required" could be a short time. On the other hand, the stuff of real life is complicated, and the "mental problems" brought to psychiatry and psychotherapy are always entwined with problems in living. Even when troubles in relating to self and to others arise suddenly in response to situational stress, it can take some time for a person to dare to explore with another person the disturbing impact of what's happening, and thus come to understand and feel it differently.

Nor is it surprising that effective psychotherapy takes years, not months, with people who have suffered significant relational trauma at critical times in their lives, leaving them with unexamined, deeply held convictions that interpersonal connection is stressful or dangerous, that others are malevolent or indifferent in relation to an essentially alien or worthless self. These are the sorts of emotional convictions that underlie and generate chronic anger, depression, anxiety, self-harm, hostility, addiction, superiority, hypervigilance, dissociation, volatility, suicidality, relational instability and more – a whole gamut of symptoms that turn up as markers of various disorders in the DSM-5 (American Psychiatric Association, 2013).

When one's experience is that relationships cause stress and pain, whether through familial abuse and neglect or through societal misrecognition and marginalization (or both), it's a long-term project just to come to trust a relationship in which one's experience is taken seriously. From a position of social and/or psychological vulnerability, it takes courage to be emotionally vulnerable. And then there's the work of self-understanding and finding out how one's relational experience with others can change. Such psychotherapy often requires a long-term investment of time and energy.

Why would this be a bad thing? In other aspects of life, sustained effort to change personal patterns is seen as courageous commitment. One might do weekly physical training or yoga classes for a very long time to undo the destructive habits of a lifetime. Likewise, psychotherapy could be sprung free from a medical-model focus on symptom relief and released into interaction with whole persons who live complex lives and strive to find mental/emotional well-being in the midst of challenging circumstances.

But could this "emancipated" psychotherapy – a steady, helpful relationship that's available to people for as long as they choose to come – get funded within medical and insurance systems that are organized around disorder, diagnosis, and symptom relief? Probably not. This has become another case of "the rich get richer." Those who can afford to pay for services have access to better lives in many ways; being able to afford long-term, non-pathologizing psychotherapy is one of them.

Sometimes societies collectively decide that their members should be supported to receive certain services, from garbage collection to secondary education to basic health care. Whyever not support access to psychotherapy for those who want and need it? The program would pay for itself not only in direct social benefits, but also financially, reducing the incidence of acute "mental illness" and stress-related physical illness and all the associated costs for treatment. A paradigm of prevention and wellness is good for societies as well as for individuals. Unfortunately, however, a paradigm of treating disease is easier to understand and to practice.

Nevertheless, relational psychotherapists carry on with practice oriented to interpersonal connection and subjective wellness. Our alternative point of view is not wrong just because it's a minority view. In fact, specific intersubjective factors of relational therapy practice could probably be shown to be mutative, if there were the political and scientific will to design such studies.

On the other hand, perhaps it's for good reason that relational practice resists being "objectified," that we find our evidence-base in conversations with clients and colleagues, that instead of designing quantitative studies, we tell subjective and intersubjective stories (a long, strong tradition in psychoanalytic writing). In any case, that's what I will do here: tell the story of a therapy that has put into practice the alternative assumptions I have outlined, a therapy that for inherent relational reasons could only have been long-term.

My clinical perspective

First let me introduce myself as a clinician. In 30 years of general practice as a social worker and psychotherapist, I have found that relational psychotherapy can be effective over a short span of sessions, and that it can also sustain a very long trajectory of major growth and change. In either case, I offer talk therapy with the goal of "making sense together" (Buirski & Haglund, 2009).

In my short-term work with clients, we explore thoughts and emotions, note relationship patterns, highlight personal strengths, reframe problems, ease shame, and bolster agency in relationship to self and others. In longer-term work, we do more of the same, but in clinical consultation on the work, I might use language about insecure attachment, about making contact with frightened and persecutory parts of self, about containing affect to ease dissociative splitting, about enactments of repetitive and self-object transference, or about the process of a fragmented self becoming more cohesive, self-aware, resilient, enlivened, and connected with others.

These are my clinical languages, both everyday and technical. But I often remind myself that what I offer to any client is simply (and not so simply) a special form of listening. The language for it might go something like this: *I will be with you – listen and respond to you – with focused, steady empathy, respectful curiosity, and the intention to understand you from within your experience. This may allow you to be with yourself differently – with more self-respect and self-understanding – and be with other people differently, too.*

I needed this simple mantra to ground my work with James, because for years the sense we were making together was as opaque to me as James's subjective emotional experience, obscured rather than revealed by his words. He often noted that his mother, a psychoanalyst, told him that his therapy should be about his subjectivity. Just as often, in full discursive, expository mode, he would hold up a finger to stop any (mother-like) interference from me and say, "I know what I'm doing."

My own theory told me to trust that James's psychological, emotional, and relational systems would use me wisely, but sometimes I "trusted" only because I couldn't think of an alternative. And yet, as it turns out, he did know what he was doing.

James

James was 36 years old when he read the first edition of my text on relational psychotherapy, just released (DeYoung, 2003), and then called for an appointment. He came ten times over ten months before he asked for weekly sessions, which lasted another ten months. Then he settled into a steady routine of three sessions a week for more than eight years. Five years ago, he decided he could manage with two sessions a week, and that's our current pattern. Over 15 years, we have spent around 1,600 50-minute sessions together.

James is a client whom medically minded therapists would have felt duty bound to diagnose and medicate. In fact, he had been both diagnosed and medicated in his mid-twenties. "Mental Health System" words like *schizophrenia* and *psychosis* felt to him like deep misunderstanding, collusion, and torture. I never heard what medications had been tried or why he was now off medication, and I decided, since it was clear to me that he was not a danger to himself or others, that I didn't need to know. To ask would have been an objectifying impingement, and it seemed to me that such impingement was the enemy.

James was fortunate that his parents were willing to divert funds "for later when we're gone" into treatment that might give their son a better life here and now. James could appreciate psychotherapy as a non-medical process because he understood that this was the kind of work done by his mother, his main support in life. It was clear early on that James didn't experience my professional connections with his mother as an impingement, but rather as assurance of my trustworthiness.

What might happen for someone with an atypical, currently fragmented, highly pathologized self-system when a therapist offers a non-pathologizing relational paradigm of treatment, and the client is given the opportunity to work within that paradigm for as long as it takes? All three of us – James, his mother, and I – have been tenaciously committed to testing that question. But the therapy has belonged entirely to James. He has made sure of that.

The trouble

James grew up in comfortable circumstances: white, urban, upper middle-class; his adult role models were professionals and corporate executives. His parents separated when he was ten, and he and his two sisters lived mostly with his mother with regular contact with their father. Heterosexual and cisgender, he had several girlfriends before his breakdown. Exceptionally able-bodied, he once cycled across Canada, and still goes for long runs several times a week. He did well in school until the assault that took out his right eye at 16, and then a transfer to a small alternative high school seemed to settle him. He won a provincial scholarship for his art portfolio, went to art college and graduated successfully.

After a stint studying painting in Italy, James came home to begin adult life. He often says that he had assumed that it would somehow just unfold for him the way it had for his parents: Life is set up so that you get a job, then a wife, a house, and kids. There was no such structure into which he could step, so he improvised. He had an apartment with a roommate, then with a girlfriend. He rented a studio where he could both live and paint and also teach painting sometimes. He supported himself with steady work as a theater usher.

But things started to fall apart. It's no accident that I have no clear picture of how the breakdown progressed or for how long. James's memories of this time are fragments with no sequence: running from a restaurant in terror of the friends he had been sitting with; throwing all of his art into a dumpster; sitting in his father's basement after losing his studio and feeling the universe expanding into awful nothingness above him; concerns about the occult, the Mafia, the collusion of evil powers in the world, pressing concerns that took up all of his mental space. His father tried to help by giving him a place to stay and finding him janitorial work. Meanwhile, James's mother went through radical cancer treatment, a shocking scare that has just lately become located in time for him. Someone took him to a mental health facility where a psychiatrist treated him as if he were defective and prescribed him medication. For a time he lived in a hostel at night and on the street in the daytime.

By the time James came to me, his life had been restructured. On a government disability support program, he lived alone in an apartment, and he worked several shifts a week in a café set up to give people with mental health challenges a place to practice work-skills. But he was haunted by what the breakdown had done to him – as if he had awoken from a nightmare, but awoken changed by the nightmare into something he had never been; he mentioned Kafka's cockroach. He could not be this destitute mental patient who had lived in a hostel with homeless men and shared downtown streets with society's losers. It was not the life he had thought would be his: alone, and being treated like scum, like garbage.

As I began work with James it was clear that I needed a clinical point of view that would take seriously his experience of catastrophe while also not treating him (however inadvertently) like "a walking defect, a piece of garbage." I found what I needed in Atwood's inquiry into extreme states of self-fragmentation, self-loss and self-annihilation – an inquiry that covers what traditional psychopathology calls psychosis, but from a non-medical, phenomenological point of view (Atwood, 1997). Such states are the result, Atwood maintained, "of an intersubjective catastrophe in which psychologically sustaining relations to the human surround have broken down at their most basic level" (p. 55). It seemed to me that although James's material existence had become stable and safe, he was living within that relational catastrophe every day. Atwood suggested that the catastrophe of self-loss will continue for as long as the patient experiences extreme vulnerability and a need for archaic validation that is met by misunderstanding, objectification, and invalidation. Often such patients can communicate their experience only in concretized forms – delusions, hallucinations, and enactments.

What some might call delusions, James called his "concerns." When he spoke of them directly – for example, that someone would come up on his blind side on the street and shoot him in the head with a 48 pistol – he would qualify their truth value: "I'm not saying that's *going* to happen. I'm just saying it could. It *could* happen, right? You can't say it's impossible." It was essential that I agree with his argument. For my own sake (and his?) I also sometimes needed to say that I thought it wouldn't be likely. I might sometimes add that I knew he had already been blindsided by a violent hit to the head, that the world can for sure be a dangerous place.

In similar fashion, when responding to his ideas about past events – for example, that there had been a highly choreographed plot to take out his eye, or that someone had sprayed an aerosol or slipped LSD into his eye socket to alter his brain – it was important for me not to contradict his theories, but rather to take them in (not interpret them) as face-value metaphors for being wiped out by forces he could not defend against or even recognize. A list of such concerns was always available, and one of them would come up when for some reason James was feeling especially vulnerable. Sometimes I could guess at the reason, the extra vulnerability, but it was not helpful for me to suggest a connection between his feeling vulnerable and his concerns.

Many of James's concerns during the early years of our work weren't put in such directly personal terms, though they hinted at personal anxieties. He was very disturbed by the idea of snuff films, by thoughts of crooked, brutal cops, by the sadisms and tortures let loose in the world through the hidden collusions of politicians and the Mafia, for example. He found relief from such upsetting concerns by shifting to preoccupations about artists and the making of art. Carrying his early love of fresco painting forward, he would spend weeks thinking, for example, about the place of eggs in creating artistic surfaces, many session hours describing his artistic experiments that followed on what Da Vinci and Michelangelo must have been trying to figure out. Maybe they tried painting on an egg and wheat surface … on lasagna noodles. It was *possible*. I had to agree.

As we continued into the middle years of therapy, James noticed that his concerns were fading. I noticed that his novel artistic ideas were becoming more achievable. I can hypothesize that this shift happened as James's sense of interpersonal vulnerability and his need for archaic validation (a validation of feeling, not of logic) were met again and again not by misunderstanding, objectification, and invalidation but by understanding and acceptance. As James's concerns diminished, he was able to shift into more direct expression of what the trouble was.

The therapy conversation

I can't, however, speak of "more direct expression" without clarifying the nature of our conversations. Even as his concerns have diminished, James has remained a master of circumlocution – as if speaking personal emotional truth would explode his world. I can understand that if his breakdown were an experience of intense affect made unbearable by intersubjective failures of understanding, his system would protect him from doing anything to recreate that situation. At the same time, I can understand him, as his mother does now, as a person with Asperger's syndrome – and if so, how much more likely those intersubjective failures of understanding would be, especially at times of high stress.

James has let me know that *autistic* is a mental health word, like *schizophrenic*, which he finds dehumanizing and demeaning. We haven't spoken of either word in relation to him. I think he knows that I don't use labels for people, and that I accept that his brain works the way that it does. I appreciate the reality of neurodiversity – by definition a spectrum of difference, not of pathology. What matters is that this person who is uniquely James, with his differences, finds a place of satisfaction and well-being in life. What helps us in our psychotherapy project is finding a way to communicate that works for us.

And so, in his way of communicating, James has come to every session with topics to talk about, intent on having his meanings understood, on having the *experience* of being understood. My job has been to understand each narrative or explanation moment to moment, step by step. He is not hard to follow; he explains each new term as he proceeds. In lecture mode, his voice comes at me in monotone, and as I fight to hear the person behind the articulate verbosity, I sometimes fight sleep. This happens as he explains Sharia law, the custom of hajj, Tibetan Buddhism, the relationship of Krishna and Arjuna on the Bhagavad Gita battlefield. It happens as he contrasts Canadian and American ways of treating people, the different rules for life in democracies and police states, the different measures by which people become George W. Bush or a loser.

These and many other repeated topics are not random; they weave an associational web of meaning around significant events and desires in James's life. Wearing his difference and seeking identity, an adolescent James dressed "East Indian" and read the *Tao Te Ching*. The young man who smashed a beer bottle into James's eye was from Pakistan, assumed Muslim. In the extremity of James's breakdown suffering, he found daily refuge in a temple where a Korean Buddhist monk taught him to meditate and gave him a koan along with simple tasks in the temple community. He once went with his mother to hear the Dalai Lama speak, reveres him as His Holiness, and seeks to follow his teachings. Following teachings gives one's life purposeful structure, even when the going is very hard. This is Krishna's lesson for Arjuna, and what a hajj journey enacts.

The relationship between James, the wandering artist who talks in metaphor, and his father, the corporate executive who makes money and talks sense, has been difficult for many years. In states of intense concern,

James associates his father with gun violence (there's a history of duck hunting and skeet shooting together) and brutal, depersonalizing American values (his father has US citizenship). The relationship between James and his social world is often a question of getting the rules right. He wants to live life on his own terms, but he can't bear being in trouble. Once, during his years of walking the streets, he was arrested and held in jail on suspicions that proved groundless. Now the appearance of a police officer on the street terrifies him. Why does George W. Bush matter? I believe he embodies for James what a person can become – what James could have become, as their faces are similar – when everything goes as it should, and a life of power and success is handed from American father to son.

It doesn't matter to James that I see connections between such topics and his life experience. What matters is that I listen and follow each time he retraces a section of the tapestry. After five years of conversation that moved between concerns about sadistic violence, possible surfaces on which to paint, and explanations of sociocultural topics, another kind of conversation emerged among his topics. He began to be consistently angry about his life. I did not find myself sleepy.

But even then he spoke "objectively," focusing his rage on the garbagy, bag-of-shit, scum people who have made his life hell, depriving him of his chance to have a wife and children, a house and a life, taking his eye out, driving him down and stomping on him. Sometimes the makers of beer bottles were implicated, and we agreed that thinking about blowing up beer plants made him feel a bit better. But mostly it was people who looked down on him, who squished him into nothing, that he wanted to WIPE OUT. His actual retaliation was to turn the tables of loathing on them, to describe them in the ugliest, most despicable terms he could imagine. He would follow that by reminding me of his Decision: "No entry," he would say, crossing his hands over his chest. "You get nothing from me. The door is shut." (I thought of Atwood and reclaiming an aspect of lost self by asserting a boundary against the forces that would usurp and annihilate.)

Once I made the mistake of asking who the people were who had made his life such hell, wondering if speaking of particular experiences might be helpful. I had noticed that sometimes the rage came after a shift at work, sometimes after spending time with the successful members of his family. But to ask "Who?" was an undermining question, I realized, as if I were trying to invalidate his rage about his losses. His most excruciating loss was his terrible fall from feeling beloved in his being and admired for his accomplishments to feeling like a despised and worthless piece of garbage. He saw that fall in the eyes of others again and again, even in the eyes of family members who wanted him to be different. So yes, all those eyes were causing him terrible pain; there was deep truth in his rage at them and his decision to shut the door against their intrusion.

This time of bitter, retaliatory anger lasted more than two years. But not every session was rageful. Often we would begin with the litany of bitterness on Tuesday, and two days later we would be talking mostly of other things (if only to start again bitterly on the following Tuesday). He began to describe time spent with his family, including his father, as tolerable, sometimes almost pleasant. And he threw himself into learning to play flamenco guitar. He found an open mic venue where every Wednesday night he could perform a piece or two he was working on, and every Wednesday he would turn up in therapy with his second-best, "travel" guitar. He had blown all his savings on what he described in detail as a beautiful handmade instrument, but he kept that one safe at home, never sorry for a moment about the expense of the purchase. (I thought of James as a one-of-a-kind instrument.) As he laid out for me his process of learning the forms of flamenco – including hours of repetitive practice with a metronome – I thought of the parallel between the dynamic, rhythmic energy of flamenco guitar and the rise and fall of vitality affect that, when synchronized between infant and caregiver, consolidates a core sense of self (Stern, 1985).

Self-regulation and mutual regulation

This was not the first time I had been struck by James's skill at finding physical ways to regulate his affective experience. When I first knew him, he walked miles a day. He told me that if you don't want to be caught talking to yourself on the street, what you do is call your own number on your cell and pretend to have a conversation. After we had settled into a steady three sessions per week, he bought himself a sketchbook, and he found that filling pages with pencil sketches of figures in motion made him feel calm and purposeful, an artist at work. And so he bought 50 sketchbooks, and he took one with him wherever he went. That Christmas he gave me a specially bound empty sketchbook for my own use; he told me I could use it for writing, too.

When James offered such moments of mutual connection to me, I received them with thanks. Briefly but truthfully, I answered his polite questions about my writing, my education, my father, my son, my weekend, my holiday (and so forth), understanding that my answers went into his web of meanings where I might not recognize myself. On the other hand, there was his story of a previous therapy in contrast to ours. It had failed when he couldn't get past his mistrust and anger, which he called "transference." I asked if he knew how we might keep that from happening between us. "It won't happen," he said. "You talk to me." This exchange, years ago, was a surprise, for in those days it seemed to me that James usually received my talking as an interruption. He would need several moments just to take in what I had said, and responding was effortful.

But at the non-verbal level of vitality affect, of what Schore (2012) would call right-brain regulation, we were synchronizing well enough, doing mutual regulation well enough, to allow some things to change. As noted, James became able to bring me his rage to feel, over and over. Sometimes he would tell me it wasn't *at* me. I would say, "I know it's not *at* me, and it's important to share it with me."

In terms of Schore's right-brain theory, I have thought about the activity within James's right brain – his non-linear world of visceral affect, emotion, pre-verbal apprehensions, associational meanings, relational intuitions, images, metaphor, color, texture, rhythm and melody – and I have wondered whether the firing there has always been more powerful and complex than he and would-be co-regulators could manage. Therefore, perhaps, his retreat from right-brain chaos to linear, logical left-brain explanations, with a thick wall thrown up between the two.

Yet the whole of James has been communicating despite the split, and, to use Schore's language, right-brain overstimulation and dissociation have been diminishing from the bottom up and the top down. His right brain is becoming available for co-regulated relationship. My measure of this change is the amount of time James is able to spend talking *with* me – sharing affectively nuanced relational conversation – compared to the amount of time James talks *at* me. In the early years, such genuine conversation was rare. Now we have mutual conversation in some part of every session, some days with only brief forays into highly linear explanations of topics. Meanwhile, in the last two years, James has begun to teach himself classical guitar, which he now finds surprisingly beautiful. It's the emotions in the music, he says. They aren't just the push and drive of flamenco. Even the simple pieces have depth and complexity of feeling in them, "and I never knew that."

Trauma theory

As most clients do, James is using psychotherapy to rewrite the narrative that gives his life meaning. It was progress for him to move from "I am a wandering, worthless failure" to "I am an angry victim of deliberate, demeaning torture." Now he is considering that perhaps torture isn't the right word; what happened wasn't political and maybe it wasn't even deliberate. "Getting my eye smashed out was *trauma*," he has decided. He has read about trauma. It can change your brain, make you frightened for the rest of your life. He notes that lots of people have trauma: soldiers, accident victims, victims of crime like himself. Trauma is not mental illness.

I tell him I agree: "Trauma isn't something that's wrong with you; it's something that happened to you." And while I agree, I would also expand the trauma narrative beyond what happened to him when he was 16. At 16, post-traumatic stress symptoms would have become one more set of demands on his capacity for self-regulation, his well-developed ability to push himself hard. As the supportive structures of home and schooling fell away, as his mother fell dangerously ill, as the fear of not being able to produce great art bore down on him, cumulative stress overwhelmed his system's capacity to regulate, and he "decompensated." He fell apart and lost himself – another terrifying trauma happened to him.

And then an even more devastating trauma happened. In his state of intense vulnerability, he needed the non-pathologizing, personal presence of someone who could connect in a right-brain regulating way with his deep fear and confusion. Instead he felt distanced, objectified, turned into a defective mental patient, his languages misunderstood, his experiences invalidated. This relational trauma continued as the interpersonal catastrophe within which he lived for years. This is not to blame those who tried to help, but to acknowledge the potential for destruction inherent in a mismatch between help needed and help offered, destruction experienced as assaultive trauma.

Nevertheless, as James points out, there's good news about trauma: you *can* come out the other side. It's possible. James believes this is happening for him. He is not a mental patient for life. He is a trauma survivor who is recovering.

Changes for the better

What is the nature of James's recovery? Both subtle and profound, his recovery is most evident in changes in the quality of his self-experience.

Since early days, there has been a steady increase in James's capacity to talk about his dysregulated states after they pass, especially his states of concern, incoherence ("wandering off"), and rageful anger. His most frightening concerns seem to be a thing of the past. As they faded, he talked about being able to relax – such a good surprise, he said, after years and years of being tense all the time.

James's strategies for affective self-regulation have become more complex and nuanced – from endless walking the streets and making repeated calls to organizations that seek justice for victims of violence, to practicing classical guitar and going to yoga classes to calm his nervous system.

Over the years, James has struggled mightily with his self-concept and self-esteem. He has described a world of people at the top – their success, brilliance, fame – and how he wants to be there too, not a loser, not a nothing. Part of him was on a tireless search for the brilliant unifying idea, artistic project, or musical virtuosity that would put him up there. And over the years, he slowly gave up the search, which he himself called "grandiose." He concluded, "I can't solve the problems of the universe, explain it all with a theory. I just have to make sense of my own little world, tie my shoes like everybody else, get on the subway."

For several years, James has started many sessions saying, "I'm working away at my art and my music, and I'm pleased with my progress." Recently he was talking about how people make meaningful lives. "They have partners and families," he said.

> That won't be for me; my path has been toward art instead. Finally I have one painting on my wall that I really like. There will be more, I'm pretty confident. A dozen, maybe. I don't need to be famous with 60,000 paintings. My meaning-of-life doesn't have to be big, just what's mine.

Feeling constantly threatened and intensely anxious doesn't leave much room for empathy, and so it has been only lately that James has begun to talk about what others feel. He watches the news now, and he says that what he feels for the people being bombed in Syria, for example, has changed. It used to be if he watched it, it was like it was happening to him. But now he knows, "It's their lives, not mine. They are suffering and dying. There's a lot of pain in the world. A lot of people hurt." Closer to home he noticed that a fellow who works at the café with him just keeps getting beaten down by life. "I feel sorry for the little guy."

Gratitude and softer qualities of memory have become available to James. Reminiscing about the Korean Buddhist monk who gave him shelter, James remarked, "He gave me a lot. Maybe he saved my life. That was kindness." He told his mother that he was thinking about how nice it was, when he was a kid, for his aunt and uncle to take him along with his cousins on cycling and camping trips. Sharing this conversation with me, he commented, "It's weird. I use to think it was all bad, people were always all against me. But my aunt and uncle were generous. Now I think it was just *some* bad people putting me down *some* of the time." Then quietly, an afterthought: "I don't even know who they are." (I wondered who "internal bad objects" are when they're not being projected.)

Socializing remains difficult for James. As he puts it,

> Me with myself, that's pretty good now. Me and other people, still not so good. I've got a lot to learn. Like sometimes people don't want to hear you go on about something, even if it's really interesting to you.

He has found a Tibetan coffee shop where he works on his sketchbooks and chats with staff. He did a portrait of the Dalai Lama for one of them, who later gave him a shirt and some prayer beads that she said came from her home village, from someone who had once been a teacher to the Dalai Lama.

He says he is working this through.

> You know how people have stories about their lives and there's a turning point? I'm not going to question my luck to be given these things. Maybe this is a turning point and I don't have to feel like such a shmuck anymore.

Meanwhile he has taken up yoga, and for him the best part, after years of being identified with groups of "people with difficulties" is being just a person in a group of people who like yoga and are doing it together. "The teacher was really nice to me, walked out with me after. Chatted. I didn't know what to do. After all those years of feeling like something people scrape off their shoe."

Changes between us

Changes in James's sense of self have changed the quality of our relationship, and vice versa, chicken-and-egg. We converse. He can say "I" and "you." We are more relaxed together. Our connection can hold more trouble. One session he picked a fight with me, firing questions to prove points. I pushed back a bit, and the anger dissolved as he told me details of what he remembered from the night he lost his eye. Then he wanted to clarify, "So you've never been physically damaged and had a loss like that?" I said no. "Emotionally damaged?" I said yes. "How?" I told him I felt that was private. "I understand that," he replied. On his way out he told me I had done good work that day.

A month later, when I had asked him to come in an hour early so that I could get to a medical appointment, he arrived hostile again. "Will people at work think that because I left early I'm in a mental health crisis?" He popped out his prosthetic eye and laid it carefully on the coffee table between us. "Is that something made by Ford? Technology kills." Then he was off on his old rant about sadistic people everywhere, no friendliness anywhere in his life. Nearing the end of the session, he stopped, put his eye back in, and said in a different tone, "So do you sometimes have a really bad day, feel totally out of sorts, and you just have to push yourself through it?" I told him that yes, indeed, sometimes that happened to me.

The next session he asked if I had been confused when he took his eye out (I had been confused; it had been a first). He explained that taking his eye out and putting it back in helps shift something for him. Also, it's very clear evidence that it's true: the loss. I said that it had made the loss very clear to me.

When I asked James for permission to write about our work together, I told him I would like for him to read it, and I wouldn't publish anything he wasn't okay with. He said yes immediately – and so I knew to keep listening. In the next session he told me his mom thought it would be safe. He also mentioned that lately people have come to understand that people can have a disability and also have strengths … that someone might agree or disagree with my professional knowledge … that maybe an organization of therapists is like the Mafia. I answered each of his implicit questions as directly as I could. Two days later he came directly to the point: "About including me in your writing … So you know I have trust issues."

"Yes, I do know that."

"And that's not unusual."

"No, it's not unusual."

"There's an issue with favourable and unfavourable. The power of that takes over, separates people. If you're seen favourably, you get a favourable life; if you're seen unfavourably, you get an unfavourable life … Countries make legislation to control this, to control exclusion … You're a psychologist, a different kind of entity, not religious, not political. A different kind of making space."

"I hope so," I said.

He left cheerfully. "Good talking to you!" But I wasn't sure the issue was resolved. A week later, he mentioned that his mother and I are on good terms and that Canada and the US have different approaches to personal security. I wondered out loud if maybe he was concerned about personal security because I had asked to write about him. I reiterated that I would protect his identity, that he'd have the writing to read and think about and veto if he wanted. He acknowledged some concern, but pointed out that he understands the principle of common exchange.

"I have sat for a portrait before. Artists do that for each other."

I felt I had consent. Now I had to do my part to produce a draft for him to read, "a fair likeness."

Conclusion

James's ways of processing and communicating information are not average or expectable, but they have needed to be understood, not changed. His acute symptoms of distress, the fragmentation, dysregulation, and intense anxiety that made him even less accessible, have come not from his neurological difference but from his profound isolation. When James can feel that he is welcome and matters just as he is, he can connect with others. When he can connect, he feels that he matters. I believe that we all depend on that cycle for our personhood and well-being.

James's therapy continues. Will it ever finish? (Why would the question matter?) For many years, when I went on holiday, James saw my colleague down the hall, who shared my sense of James and his journey. She retired last spring, and last summer he managed a break with no one to fill in. This summer, when I told him of my upcoming two weeks of holiday, he was quiet for a long moment. Then he said, "That's okay. I have my yoga now." That's how I imagine the possibility of ending: when James feels psychologically sustained by his "human surround," when that security has held for long enough, catastrophe will no longer loom, and he will be able to move on from his therapy into other connections and pursuits that are uniquely James.

This is not a story of cure. Our therapy was never based on the assumption that there was something biologically or psychologically wrong with James that needed to be fixed or managed – the assumptions embedded in the diagnosis and treatment he was given at the time of his breakdown.[1]

I told this story to show how one might work from alternative assumptions, namely: The value of persons lies in their subjective being. Whether persons' modes of being are typical or atypical, they deserve to seek the experiences and define the meaning of their own well-being for themselves. Disordered relationships between self and social world are the most likely causes of emotional distress and ensuing psychological dysfunction. Assessment should explore clients' subjective experiences of distress in the context of their life situations – how that distress impacts their capacities for emotional and cognitive coherence, self-reflection, agency, and meaningful connection with others. Medication should be given only in the context of conversation that listens to clients' narratives. The success of therapy should be measured by clients' experiences of feeling more well, whole, and strong in themselves, and also more able to be with others comfortably, more confident of their own inherent worth in relationship.

As I have said, it doesn't follow from these assumptions that therapy be short or long, continuous or sporadic, or use the language of any particular theory. But it should be the length and approach that best helps a client recover a sense of worth and well-being in relation to self and others. If, as if often the case, that stipulation suggests longer-term therapy, *whyever not?*

We could, of course, circle back to the question of cost. James has been privileged in the support his parents can give him. Many survivors of relational trauma, employed or not, insured or not, do not have access to treatment that will help them in recovery, and the most vulnerable of them are the least likely to get the help they need. Why would it be, in affluent societies that spend billions on health care, that such preventative, restorative, humane treatment is not made widely available? The answer lies in what we as societies choose to value, in how we define being persons and being well. The answer to *whyever not?* lies in systems of belief, taken as truth; it lies in assumptions, taken as facts, which can be challenged – as James has quietly and steadfastly challenged the systems that would dehumanize and demean him.

Note

1 For evocative, challenging exploration of concepts such as *normal* and *cure*, see Eli Clare (2017), *Brilliant imperfection: Grappling with cure.*

References

American Psychiatric Association (2013). *Diagnostic and statistical manual of mental disorders* (5th ed.). Washington, DC: Author.

Atwood, G. (1997). Contexts of nonbeing: Varieties of the experience of personal annihilation. In Orange, D., Atwood, G., & Stolorow, R. (eds.), *Working intersubjectively: Contextualism in psychoanalytic practice*, pp. 45–66. Hillsdale, NJ: Analytic Press.

Buirski, B. & Haglund, P. (2009). *Making sense together: The intersubjective approach to psychotherapy.* New York: Jason Aronson.
Clare, E. (2017). *Brilliant imperfection: Grappling with cure.* Durham, NC: Duke University Press.
DeYoung, P. (2003). *Relational psychotherapy: A primer.* New York: Routledge.
Schore, A. (2012). *The science of the art of psychotherapy.* New York: W. W. Norton.
Stern, D.N. (1985). *The interpersonal world of the infant.* New York: HarperCollins.

Chapter 3

It takes as long as it takes

Therapists' subjective experiences of long-term therapy

Jean Kotcher

Is long-term treatment (15 or more years), "Frozen time and endless analyses" (Dragosei, 2007)? Angela Connolly Dragosei searingly critiqued David Tresan's (2007a) endorsement of long-term analysis. She asserted that when treatment continues open-endedly, the analytic pair is frozen in futile and indefinite waiting. Tresan (2007b), in a heated rebuttal, stated that long-term work is a mode of treatment that has existed and been ignored for a long time by all analytic schools: "Far from being frozen, these patients are the most supple I know" (p. 49). Likewise, Warren Poland (1997) objected to depictions of long-term analyses that implied stalemate or exploitation, "as if the only real question were whether the practicing analyst were stupid or, instead, a knave" (p. 184). This chapter explores the controversy in psychoanalytic thinking on long-term treatment and makes a case for its clinical value, offering the results of a study I conducted on long-term therapy in 2012.

Very long-term therapies have conceptually entered a kind of no man's land that does not have adequate road maps. In fact, there has been a dearth of professional literature or discussion on the value of long-term treatment. Analytic therapists tend to not talk about their long-term cases except in select and trusted settings. It's as if there is such great ambivalence that a gag order has been placed on this topic, which is part of the clinical life of many therapists. I myself fell under this taboo and realized my own ambivalence toward discussing the work with long-term patients I was seeing. This was curious, as these cases were among the most interesting in the clinical work in which I was engaged. I began to want to know more about how other therapists who conducted long-term therapies thought and felt about their work.

My interest led me to conduct a qualitative study (Kotcher, 2012) in which I interviewed seven San Francisco Bay Area psychoanalytically oriented therapists. My primary goal was for these experienced and highly regarded clinicians to speak about their experiences and contribute to the discussion using their own voices. Also central were questions about how they thought about long-term cases in relation to the concept of termination, and what theoretical concepts guided them about the nature of the long-term therapy relationship and the course of treatment. Doidge et al. (2002) designated long-term psychoanalysis on average as lasting six years in the US, Canada and Australia. I chose 15 years as the definition of a long-term treatment for my study because it stands in such contrast to therapists' experience of treatments that last six, or even, ten years.

I begin with two clinical examples from my own work, highlighting long-term therapy aspects of the cases. The first is a case in which psychological and life problems remain in the foreground of our ongoing work. In the second, my patient chose to continue treatment after issues that brought her to therapy had subsided. The case examples are followed by a discussion of several of the more important findings from my study, including a suggestion of a developmental road map for long-term therapy.

You're on your own—Peter

Peter told me in our first session, "When I found out I was HIV-positive, I made up my mind it was not going to be a death sentence for me." He also shared his mental image of patrolling a fence around land to make sure there were no holes that needed repair. Though for Peter the image of patrolling a guarded estate to keep it secure referred to his HIV status, there was much more to the story. I had a sense that he wanted to confront the early developmental failures that prevented him from taking on life more fully, but he felt a deep need to keep himself protected from disappointments by others. This made our work have a quality of being stilted or frozen, followed by small incremental periods of growth and integration, and of owning his right to take risks. With his need to survive being HIV-positive, it took time and energy for him to manage his medical situation which was ever present in our work. Only in the last six years was Peter able to put his status in the background and separate the past from the present struggles he has in relating to others. In retrospect, it makes sense that our work together has been over 28 years.

I told Peter that I wanted to include our work together in this chapter and he asked me to write about what it has been like for him to live with HIV. It caused him to put his life "on hold" in so many ways.

Toward the end of his first year of therapy, Peter was fired from work and took a hiatus from treatment. Months passed when I did not hear from him and I began to worry, so I called him. He told me he had just found out that his T-cell count had fallen close to an AIDS diagnosis. He returned to therapy immediately saying he wanted me to be part of his "HIV team." Over time after returning to therapy, his T-cell count returned to a high level and his HIV viral load became undetectable. Though Peter has always followed his medication and personal regimens (he doesn't drink or use drugs and goes to the gym almost daily), our work together gave him the emotional foundation to ensure that his anxiety and despair were lifted. This was the first time that Peter had let down his fence to let another person help him emotionally.

Peter and his (non-biological) brother were adopted overseas when they were both three months old. He also had a sister, 18 years older, from his mother's previous, abusive marriage. His childhood was fraught with worry about his parents' chronic alcoholism and his mother's narcissistic needs and moods. He learned that his best defense was to hide problems from his parents. When he struggled academically in elementary school years, he stole test answers from teachers' desks and convinced them all that he was doing well. He hid from bullies who targeted him in middle school for seeming gay, and he dissociated when in early adolescence his mother would come into his room at night intoxicated, lay across him, and complain how men in her life had treated her. When he was 18, his parents discovered he was dating a man—his mother threw him out and his father told him, "You're on your own now." He moved from the East Coast to San Francisco and put himself through art school, keeping in contact with his parents and occasionally flying to the East Coast to see them. He and his family never again referred to his sexuality and he never told his parents he was HIV-positive. When his mother died, a few years after his father, she left her entire estate to Peter's brother who had remained in the same town, was married, and had two children. She left nothing to Peter or his sister who had both moved away and were both gay.

Though Peter is handsome and has a cheerful demeanor and creative and thoughtful internal life, one can see from his history that he had every reason to not trust others and remain guarded. On the one hand, Peter's and my work together has felt close and caring. On the other hand, there have been issues he lived with that took a long time for him to uncover. For example, it was seven or eight years before he told me about his nightmares of murderous creatures hiding in his closet causing him to switch on the light in panic and search the closet and room to reassure himself there was nothing there. It took many years for him to begin to process the depths of fear he had about HIV and to grieve the loss of friends and acquaintances. This has progressed over the years at a pace and manner that is right for him. As the years passed and Peter was able to take more risks (such as taking speech and acting classes), he was able to let down his guard more with others. This was a major accomplishment, as one of the most elusive aspects of our work together has been his being more open and expressive with others. I asked him if he wished he had taken these classes before and he told me, "I don't think I had come to it yet. I wasn't ready until now."

As slowly as needed—Ella

In contrast to my work with Peter, Ella and I were involved in a powerful process, starting 32 years ago, which was slow and progressive. She initiated therapy after being unexpectedly "dumped" by her boyfriend, which precipitated her going to the Golden Gate Bridge where friends convinced her not to jump. Her suicidal behavior made sense, as she had lost her mooring at the age of 12 when her mother died of cancer. Ella grew up in a working-class family in the Midwest with parents who had "hair-trigger tempers" and disciplined her and her younger sister by hitting them with their hands, a hairbrush or belt. At the same time, her mother was nurturing and supportive of her academic achievements, resulting in Ella's being very attached to her mom. Though her mother's death was an enormous, life-altering loss to the entire family, shockingly, three months after the mother's death, the father married a woman who was selfish and cruel to Ella and her sister. As a result, their grief was suppressed. Ella told me in our second session that talking about the loss of her mother led her to have suicidal thoughts and to cut herself. The pattern was clear to me at that point; rupture and death were deeply connected and the treatment was going to have to move slowly so as not to trigger self-harming behaviors. I assured her that we could move as slowly as she needed to talk about her life.

Ella was indeed challenging. She made it clear from the beginning she wouldn't tolerate "psychobabble," was fiercely invested in her personal identity and did not want therapy to make her "a normal," like me. She and her friends were part of an art community in San Francisco who mistrusted government and sometimes each other, leading to volatile conflicts that occasionally became physical. She could be volcanic in our sessions, either containing eruptions or spilling over as she railed about painful episodes with friends. At other times, she would sit through half or more of a session, not speaking, with her eyes closed and her head turned away from me. I felt helpless about how to respond to her varied and dysregulated states. She reported her parents complained that she was inconsolable as a baby and young child because she did not like being held. Eventually, during silences, I began to talk softly and slowly about what I imagined she could be feeling. This went on for months until she began to correct me, wanting me to know that her episodes of "shutting down" were sometimes reactions to something I had said in the current or previous session. This felt like the beginning of trust in our relationship.

Our sessions increasingly provided emotional regulation that had been missing in Ella's development. She eventually began to talk with me about her family's intergenerational abuse and the underlying causes of her dysregulation—her mother and aunts were sexually abused by their father. Ella's father suffered from untreated PTSD from combat in World War II, and two of her maternal cousins committed suicide in their teens.

Over time she used the therapy to monitor her own depression and suicidal thoughts, and her urge to "shut down." She had a few short-lived abusive relationships that ended badly. Subsequently, she entered a seven-year relationship with a man that was initially gratifying. However, with time he grew psychologically unstable, becoming overly dependent on her, and the relationship deteriorated. She and I discussed the relationship extensively and eventually she grew so frustrated with the disparities between her developing internal strengths and his instability that she ended it with no need to harm herself. At around that time, she turned her attention to developing stable and meaningful friendships that have since flourished. Finally, the deep connection between endings and death was broken.

Further evidence of Ella's internal growth is that when her father died ten years ago, she felt his loss deeply and was able to take her time and grieve with me. Several years earlier, after her stepmother's death, she had been able to reconnect with her father and they created a rich and empathic relationship. Over the years, she had also returned to her interrupted process of mourning the loss of her mother, reclaiming aspects of her positive identification with her mom that are part of her own strengths.

It was around five years ago that I wondered if Ella might be ready to end her therapy. I realized that she had grown comfortable owning her own strengths, creativity and accomplishments, something that had been previously denied her. Naturally, over the 32 years of therapy, a positive mutual regard and sharing of overlapping interests has developed. We have come to feel a strong affection for each other and appreciate our shared interests in politics and the arts. This development in the therapy has been quite therapeutic, enhancing Ella's confidence and sense of groundedness in her identity. I found she was also thinking about when she might feel ready to end when she raised the issue, which paved the way for us to talk more deeply about what our work has meant to both of us. Through our discussions Ella has realized that she wants to continue to see me until she retires and relocates. We've continued to pay the usual attention to her internal life and its further development with attention to how her life will change without having me and her friends here to talk to when she moves within a year.

When I told her I was writing a chapter about long-term therapy she immediately said that I needed to include our work together. I asked her what she thought about being in therapy for so long and she responded without hesitation, "I've needed it." She reminded me of the emotional turmoil some of her family members continue to live with who, unlike her, have not had decades of therapy. She has referred to them as her "control group." Ella has taken the years she "needed" to transform her own turbulent feelings. She has grown to manage differences between herself and others with wisdom and empathy, and views the state of the world and politics with resilience, even humor. From my perspective, she is an example of Tresan's (2007b) supple patient.

What the study revealed

The study participants (four women and three men) identified with a variety of psychoanalytic theories in their work: relational, object relations, intersubjective, Jungian, and attachment theory. Regardless of their psychoanalytic leanings, each supported the provision of a process that allowed people to remain in therapy as long as needed. They did not believe six, or even ten, years was enough time *for some patients* to accomplish their individual therapeutic potentials. Authors who endorse long-term treatment portray long-term therapists having patience and self-esteem that does not rely upon a timely "cure" (Bergmann, 2005), comfort with uncertainty (Poland, 1997; Shane, 2009), and an ability to commit to and be energized by long, mutually caring professional relationships, sometimes for decades (Tresan, 2007a).

One of my participants talked about being a person who "seeks the deeper realms, which is why I probably ended up doing this work." Another referred to colleagues who don't want to work long-term. She said: "I've heard analysts who say that they don't like working with people who get too dependent on them." Robert Wallerstein (1986) suggested that patients who needed long-term therapy and therapists who were comfortable working long-term tended to find each other.

Essentially, participants did not focus on preconceived theoretical concepts when talking about ongoing therapy, but demonstrated that they were guided mainly by their clinical experiences based on each patient's unique process. Interestingly, termination was the concept that represented the most discrepancy between clinicians. Although everyone recognized that all treatments inevitably end, one participant emphatically opposed termination as a preconceived phase, arguing that it felt manufactured to her. Two considered it to be an important phase of treatment with most of their cases, including long-term cases, and four acknowledged the value for some patients of dealing with loss, but did not consider it a necessary phase of treatment. All of them stated or implied that the patient was the best judge of whether they stayed or ended their therapy.

Some characteristics of long-term patients

According to my participants, all long-term patients shared a history of early childhood experiences of trauma, loss, neglect, and/or relationship deficits. Two types of patients were particularly identified: those who were continuing to work on ongoing difficult psychological and life problems, and a second group whose symptoms had abated. This latter group chose to stay in treatment to enhance further self-growth within a trusted and nurturing relationship. One participant discussed a dysregulated patient of 19 years, saying, "He just feels safe, knowing I'm with him." Another participant described a patient of 20 years whose symptoms had abated, as having "quite a successful life," being compassionate toward others, and able to be "quite a good mother," aspects that had been missing in her early history. Similarly, another participant told me about a successful artist patient with a happy marriage and many good friends, who had been in therapy with her for 17 years. He was not a person who opened up easily to others and he wanted to continue "to talk about his inner world," even though he was moving away and would be driving quite a bit further to continue his therapy.

A developmental perspective

There are obvious parallels between the psychic development that occurs during the course of long-term treatment and elements of actual child development—it takes at least 15 years and longer to raise a child, whether the child's development is going pretty smoothly or is challenging and uneven. Participants spoke extensively about patients who were immersed in therapeutic processes that corrected earlier developmental deficits—having a reliable, trusting relationship with a focus on their patient's needs. For those patients who did not have access to healthy emotional development earlier in life, emotional growth seemed to be the most important change they sought in therapy.

The study strongly suggested a developmental model for people to repair and rework development at a pace and manner that suited their unique needs. Participants spoke of the generally uneven pace in long-term therapy mirroring normal childhood development. "We can't move it faster," a participant emphasized, telling me that 15 years passed before her patient reached a state of trust and safety that allowed her to recall aspects of her childhood. Similarly, another said he felt that a patient was never going to "settle down" or "this was never going to end ... but the reality is that sometimes if you're patient enough things do settle down and people do start to believe that you actually are not going to betray them." In some cases, therapists can say things to patients for many years before the patient can make use of the therapist's thoughts to move forward in dealing with underlying problems. Similarly, there can be long plateaus, when nothing seems to be happening, but where time is needed to integrate the work.

This developmental perspective from the study is supported by the psychoanalytic literature. Research into early brain development emphasized that development of self-organization and self-regulation in infant development depended upon early dyadic experiences of affect regulation between parent and infant (Schore, 1994). Likewise, Hans Loewald (1960) wrote that in analysis, "the parent-child relationship can serve as a model" (p. 20). He described the parent recognizing and fulfilling needs of the infant because, at first, infants are unable to recognize or fulfill their own needs. Loewald referred to "integrative experiences" in therapy that are "comparable in their structure and significance to the early understanding between mother and child" (p. 25). His model recognizes periods of time when not much seems to be happening in long treatment and the therapist understands that the patient is integrating therapeutic experience and consolidating growth before beginning another period of activity—similar to times when a baby or child settles down and the "good-enough" parent, attuned to developmental needs, settles down with the child.

The long-term therapist's paradox

Despite their belief in the value of long-term therapy, all of my study participants voiced ethical and countertransference concerns about treatments that extended far beyond a more commonly expected time frame of approximately six years (found in the Doidge et al. report of 2002). Therapists who conduct long-term therapy tend to "hide" their long-term work from critical colleagues and feel shame about seeing someone for 15-plus years. Not only is dependency not very accepted in our culture, but even more compelling are internally driven concerns about the long-term clinical process. This was demonstrated by a participant who talked about struggles he had with a long-term patient, that things got "muddy" and "confusing", and this contributed to the long-term aspects of the case. "It seems such a difficult thing to figure whether treatment is over," he said. I was surprised to hear five participants spontaneously confess they sometimes asked themselves if another therapist might have done a better job resulting in a shorter treatment. One participant asked herself, "Is there something I'm not seeing or not doing that is making this treatment be so long?"

Though these concerns worried the participants, what they learned directly from these long-term treatments was that both patient and therapist benefited from the depth and richness of the relationships, and this served to counter their anxieties. Participants spoke about patients thriving and experiencing stability, closeness and intimacy as they went through multiple life transitions and milestones with their therapists. One observed that the people he had seen longest knew more about him than any of his other patients, though he had not necessarily disclosed more. They knew him through milestones in his life, such as births of his children and deaths of relatives, which led to a deepening of their therapeutic experience. All participants stated or implied that the therapy relationship might have been the best relationship in their long-term patients' lives. Correspondingly, these clinicians talked about their own maturational processes, growing close to patients, and being well known by them over decades. One participant talked about loving the closeness that develops in long-term therapy relationships, "I'm a person who likes a lot of intimacy. I fall in love." Another participant said, "What we shared together and what I've been to him, and what we've had together, that actually had a very profound effect on both of us."

Final thoughts

Warren Poland (1997) asked, "How long a journey should take depends on how far the destination lies. And how is one to decide that?" (p. 186). In a culture with a bias against long-term therapy, clinicians have many questions and doubts about therapy that extends far longer than they had expected. On the one hand, they understand the value of long-term treatments of 15 years or more based on direct experience with their patients that results in transformed and/or more well-regulated lives. On the other hand, long-term therapists have to contend with the hostility of colleagues, stated directly or implied, that these therapies are stalemated or, worse, examples of therapists' exploitation of their patients. Often struggling privately and having been effectively silenced, these clinicians find it difficult to discuss their long-term therapies with colleagues.

In this chapter, I have opened up a space for exploring the clinical benefits of long-term therapies. With the generosity of my research participants and of patients like Peter and Ella, I think a strong case is made for the clinical value of long-term, abiding therapies. My study and clinical cases demonstrate the following:

- Long-term patients come to treatment with a history of profound early childhood trauma, loss, neglect, and relationship deficits.
- Long-term patients often remain in therapy because of ongoing problems that can be very slow to resolve.
- Some long-term patients choose to continue their therapies, in spite of their improved lives, because they value the abiding relationship with their therapists, often the closest intimate relationship in their lives.
- Long-term treatments are often slow to start, taking a long time to develop enough safety and trust before underlying problems emerge.
- Often in these treatments, plateaus are reached where not much seems to happen, as if following a developmental road map, before growth bursts ahead.
- Long-term patients need time to rework dysfunctional attachment patterns and to mature in therapeutic relationships that can last for decades.

Perhaps the best answer to Poland's question is found in Tresan's (2007b) observation that these patients are given the unusual opportunity to relax in the care of another human being, unfreezing themselves from destructive and unsatisfying patterns and relationships, past and present, to arrive as more fully evolved people who are supple and more capable of living fuller lives. If we allow ourselves to listen and respond to the nuanced and particular developmental needs of each individual patient, we may also allow ourselves to be guided by the patient's unique process and not what the culture and some of our colleagues may be too biased or scared to consider.

References

Bergmann, M. S. (2005). Termination and reanalysis. In E. S. Person, A. M. Cooper, & G. O. Gabbard (Eds.), *Textbook of psychoanalysis* (pp. 241–253). Washington, DC: American Psychiatric Publishing.

Doidge, N., Simon, B., Brauer, L., Grant, D. C., First, M., Brunshaw, J., Lancee, W. J., Stevens, A., Oldham, J. M., & Mosher, P. (2002). Psychoanalytic patients in the U.S., Canada, and Australia: I. DSM-III-R disorders, treatment, medications, and length of treatment. *Journal of the American Psychoanalytic Association, 50*, 575–614.

Dragosei, A. C. (2007). Frozen time and endless analyses: A response to David Tresan's "Thinking individuation forward." *Journal of Analytic Psychology, 52*(1), 41–45.

Kotcher, J. (2012). *Long-term psychoanalytic psychotherapy: A study of the therapist's experience* (Unpublished doctoral dissertation). Berkeley, CA: The Sanville Institute.

Loewald, H. W. (1960). On the therapeutic action of psycho-analysis. *International Journal of Psycho-Analysis, 41*, 16–33.

Poland, W. S. (1997). On long analyses. *Psychoanalytic Psychology, 14*(2), 183–195.

Schore, A. N. (1994). *Affect regulation and the origin of the self: The neurobiology of emotional development*. Hillsdale, NJ: Lawrence Erlbaum.

Shane, E. (2009). Approaching termination: Ideal criteria versus working realities. *Psychoanalytic Inquiry, 29*, 167–173.

Tresan, D. (2007a). Thinking individuation forward. *Journal of Analytic Psychology, 52*(1), 17–40.

Tresan, D. (2007b). Time is a river without banks: A response to Connolly's "Frozen time and endless analyses." *Journal of Analytic Psychology, 52*(1), 47–49.

Wallerstein, R. S. (1986). *Forty-two lives in treatment*. New York, NY: The Guilford Press.

Chapter 4

In defense of long-term treatment

On the vanishing holding environment[1]

William S. Meyer

The mental health literature has long recognized the similarities between the role and functions of a good therapist and a good parent. Both the good therapist and the good parent are strengthened when they feel supported and diminished and made less good when their natural talents are undermined by external influences. Only recently have such impingements been inflicted on therapists; parents have been familiar with such pressures for generations.

In 1914, the US. Children's Bureau issued the first edition of the bulletin *Infant Care* (Wolfenstein, 1953). It was a compendium of bad advice. Parents were instructed to have their babies potty-trained by eight months of age. They were told that thumb-sucking and masturbation, if not rigorously interfered with, would permanently damage their child. They were warned not to pick up their crying child and that such caretaking would turn the child into a tyrant.

Many parents, particularly mothers, were torn between their own instincts and the advice of the child care experts of the day. We can sympathize and easily make allowances for those mothers who, in spite of misgivings, followed these instructions in hopes that their compliance with figures of authority would be in the best interest of their children. It is most difficult to maintain an unsupported position. It is difficult for mothers; it is difficult for clinicians.

The clinician of the 1990s is under relentless pressure to provide ever-briefer forms of treatment for all patients and clients, even though many such individuals have a compelling need for longer treatment. One recent author (Good, 1987) stated that such pressures are symptomatic of what he called "the age of Reagapeutics," in which "brief therapy is symbolic … of the modern age in which we do everything intensely and quickly" (p. 8).

These pressures abound. For instance, in a brief article titled "Finding the Right Psychotherapist" published in a widely sold consumer guide (Boardroom Classics, 1989), the first item advises consumers to look for someone who does "short-term therapy" (p. 437). Professional clinicians are tantalized by articles with sensational titles like "Psychotherapy That Takes Weeks, Not Years" (Michaels, 1989). It is telling that in my computer-generated literature review for this article, I found nearly 300 papers extolling the benefits of brief therapy and fewer than five specifically addressing its limitations.

This steady barrage of such communications cannot help but have an insidious impact on the confidence with which contemporary clinicians approach longer-term, slower-paced psychotherapy. As a consequence clinicians are at risk of caving in to outside pressures, to becoming ever-more involved in the treatment of symptoms rather than people.

How did we get to this point? The trend toward shorter relationships was noted over two decades ago in Alvin Toffler's popular book *Future Shock* (1970). He drew attention to the soaring acceleration of change in virtually all areas of contemporary society. One key symptom of this extraordinary pace, he noted, was the ascendancy of transience—the new "temporariness" in everyday life. In particular, relationships that once lasted for long periods of time had ever-decreasing life expectancies.

We can see clear evidence of such trends in mental health. In a simpler time the much-loved Harvard psychoanalyst Elvin Semrad used to tell his students, "If you want to learn about psychiatry get a good suit with two pairs of pants and be willing to sit with your patients until you have worn out the seats of both pairs of pants" (Castelnuovo-Tedesco, 1990, p. 1258). How archaic this statement seems in today's fast-paced health care market!

Bruno Bettleheim (DeAngelis, 1989) reported a seemingly minor personal incident during his training that had a profound impact on his thinking about treatment and time. At the time, Bettleheim was undergoing psychoanalysis. A disturbed young boy used to sit in the same waiting room as Bettleheim to see the wife of Bettleheim's analyst, who was one of the first child psychoanalysts. The boy, unresponsive and nearly mute, had the strange habit of plucking and chewing leaves from a cactus plant in the waiting room. As time went on Bettleheim eventually blurted out, "Johnny, I don't know how long you have been seeing Dr. X, but it must be at least two years and here you are still chewing these awful leaves" (p. 38).

Then, in Bettleheim's words,

> I still do not know how he managed to give me the impression that at this moment he was looking down at me. But he did and spoke his first sentence to me saying disdainfully, "What are two years when compared with eternity?" Johnny's comment about time permitted me to grasp that neither I nor anybody else can put a limit on the amount of time one needs to become able to cope or to change, and that trying to hurry up the process has more to do with one's own anxieties than with anything else. Only people themselves can judge when they are ready to change.
>
> (p. 38)

What has catapulted such thoughtful, patient approaches to therapeutic treatment into the hurry-up mentality of today's mental health practice?

Among many factors, none has been so influential as third-party reimbursement, a relatively recent artifact that now dominates decisions about the delivery of psychotherapeutic treatment.

From its inception psychotherapy had been financed almost exclusively in a fee-for-service two-party relationship. During the 1960s and early 1970s, however, there was rapid growth in both private and government medical health insurance plans covering treatment for psychological illnesses. As noted by Halpert (1972),

> Many of these insurance plans include partial or total reimbursement, usually up to a certain limit, for treatment in the various psychotherapies, including psychoanalysis. If the trend continues, and all indications are that it will, then even greater numbers of people will be covered for even greater total amounts for psychoanalytic treatment.
>
> (p. 122)

Practitioners of that era faced therapeutic problems that we can only wish for. In the luxury of such third-party benevolence, "The anonymous third party, the insurance company, becomes like the anonymous therapist—a transference figure. But the insurance company, unlike the therapist, *gratifies transference wishes; it takes care and protects the patient*" [emphasis added] (Halpert, 1973, p. 67). Such *was* the case in the brief Camelot era of psychotherapy reimbursement.

Contrast this with a recent report by Zuckerman (1989) on the effects of managed care on his patient, a 36-year-old, twice married, potentially abusive mother of two who presented with a long history of anxiety and depression. Zuckerman described the patient's perception of the case manager as a

> denying, ungiving mother, [and this] began to permeate her thinking. When the patient was feeling better she became afraid that the case manager, upon discovering her improvement, would feel that she was cured and withdraw his treatment authorization. When she was feeling depressed and hopeless, which was often, she felt that the case manager, upon sensing her lack of progress, would refuse to underwrite any further treatment.
>
> (p. 127)

Short-term psychotherapy

For decades, theories and methods of one or another form of brief treatment have been formulated, taught, published, and refined. And it has been repeatedly demonstrated that briefer therapies, when used appropriately, are effective.

Briefer therapies are especially useful for the basically intact person who possesses at least a modicum of ego strength, someone who, for instance, adapted reasonably well in life but became the victim of an unfortunate predicament that unduly taxed his or her endurance or rekindled a previously dormant internal conflict. Such treatment is then aimed at relieving a patient's most pressing symptoms and restoring the person to a state that existed before the acute difficulties (Castelnuovo-Tedesco, 1971).

Longer or more intensive treatment should never be invoked for trivial reasons. As Stone (1954) once pointed out,

> There is sometimes a loss of sense of proportion about the human situation, a forgetting or denial of the fact that few human beings are without some troubles, and that many must be met, if at all, by "old-fashioned" methods: courage, or wisdom, or struggle, for instance.
>
> (p. 569)

For many individuals, a few consultations or a more extended form of brief treatment is the clear treatment of choice.

Mackenzie (1991), in a comprehensive review of brief psychotherapy, defined four features requiring clinical assessment before considering a recommendation of brief psychotherapy: (1) a capacity to relate, (2) psychological mindedness, (3) motivation, and (4) evidence of adaptational strength. (For years, clinicians have acknowledged the irony that people possessing such strengths make the best use of virtually all therapeutic modalities.) Mackenzie stated that "while [the above] criteria do not in themselves constitute exclusion standards, when a patient is low on several of them, *caution should be used in recommending brief approaches*" [emphasis added] (p. 401).

As more definitive exclusion criteria, Mackenzie (1991) listed an inability to attend to the process, major characterological features that preclude effective use of the treatment, and the possibility of the patient doing harm. Included here are patients with limited impulse control, a history of repeated suicide attempts, recurrent premature termination of therapy, or entrenched alcohol or substance abuse.

Other patient characteristics Mackenzie (1991) cited that should direct clinicians' thinking away from brief therapy include the use of defenses that block access to internal states, a dominance of primitive defenses such as projection and denial, major schizoid features, major antisocial characteristics of an enduring nature, and the presence of profound negativism and rigidity. Further, Mackenzie stated that patients with a history of easily triggered suicidal ideation

> may experience the confrontational qualities of brief psychotherapy as evidence of rejection, and respond with impulsive, self-destructive behavior … Indeed when any dysfunctional characterological style is deeply pervasive and influences adaptation in many spheres of the patient's life,

> rapid alteration is not likely and a course of brief psychotherapy may be viewed by the patient as a further failure.
>
> (pp. 400–401)

Yet I recently received a postcard from an employee assistance program soliciting psychologists, social workers, and therapists to provide brief therapy for patients suffering from, among other maladies, alcoholism, chemical dependency, sequelae of sexual abuse, and eating disorders. Brief therapy, as defined by this company, was "up to four sessions."

D. W. Winnicott and the holding environment

Many elements of the therapeutic relationship, as we have known it, are reminiscent of the first relationship between infant and mother. This was first elaborated on in the eloquent writings of Donald W. Winnicott (1896–1971), an English psychoanalyst first trained as a pediatrician.

Winnicott studied and wrote extensively on the characteristics of healthy and unhealthy relationships, particularly early mother–child interactions. Winnicott was repeatedly struck by the parallels in the relationships provided by good-enough parents and those provided by successful analysts, psychotherapists, and social workers. These relationships contained common elements that facilitated development and were created by caregivers devoted to an individual's unique needs, whether the individual was a baby, a child, an analysand, a patient, or a client.

A central component of this relationship was encapsulated in Winnicott's (1965) familiar phrase, "the holding environment." Briefly, the *holding environment*, as applied to a newborn, is one that is created by a maternal figure who can identify with a baby in a state of absolute dependence and who, as needed, can provide whatever support is necessary—day and night—to meet the baby's most basic physical and psychological needs. As the infant matures, the caretaker providing the holding environment, while encouraging developmental growth, ensures that the infant is not expected to relinquish its dependent state prematurely.

A similar holding environment can be found in a therapeutic relationship. Modell (1976), while referencing psychoanalysis, makes comparisons. Like the good-enough parent, the therapist is constant and reliable, responds sensitively to the patient's affects, accepts the patient, uses judgment that is less critical and more benign, is there primarily for the patient's needs, does not retaliate, and does at times have a better grasp of the patient's inner psychic reality than does the patient and therefore can help clarify what is bewildering and confusing.

The holding environment helps to foster and does not prematurely challenge an illusion that the patient is protected from the dangers of the world and that the therapist in some way stands as a shield between the patient and these dangers. The good-enough therapist, like the good-enough parent, allows for and tolerates phase-appropriate dependency, all the while looking for opportunities to support maturational thrusts.

Holding, management, and the clinical social worker

The concept of holding at first may seem intended only for the patient suitable for analysis or insight-oriented psychotherapy. What, one may ask, of the more outwardly disturbed and challenging individual, whose treatment may require more than can be accomplished within a tidy 50-minute hour—the type of client or patient, for instance, who has traditionally been in the care of the clinical social worker?

Winnicott, who frequently lectured to social workers, expanded the concept of holding to encompass clinical management as performed by the trained psychiatric social worker. In a fine paper on case management, Kanter (1990) lamented the current perceptions of case management as an impersonal, administrative service more concerned with cutting costs than helping people in need. Winnicott, Kanter wrote, used the term "management" to describe direct interventions with the person and the environment that were aimed at facilitating the healing and maturation of even the most troubled individuals.

Winnicott elaborated on the issues of management in a personal letter (Rodman, 1987). He wrote

> In social work (as in psychoanalysis) certain factors such as reliability, dependability, and objectivity, provide a specialized environment *over a period of time* [note Winnicott's italics] in which the highly complex *internal* factors in the individual and between the various individuals in the client group may rearrange themselves. The "good" (or I would say "good enough") climate enables a client to review his or her relationship to climates that were not, or did not seem to be, good (or good enough).
>
> (p. 141)

Clinical example

I began seeing Sue nearly seven years ago. Sue was a white 35-year-old who was proud of her steady employment for the past 15 years at a nearby manufacturing plant. She was referred to me by her daughter's psychiatrist for adjunctive "parent work." Her daughter Paula, a deeply troubled adolescent, was doing miserably in relationships at home and with peers and in her school work.

Sue had divorced Paula's father shortly after Paula's birth, and she and the girl had since resided with Sue's mother. The mother, a retired woman, seemed to enjoy the secondary gain she received by virtue of her continual state of seemingly poor health.

Our initial appointment was memorable, if only for Sue's severe level of agitation. In the session she avoided eye contact, was fidgety, chain-smoked, paced, and nonverbally conveyed her terrible anxiety. As she spoke, taking quick gasps of air between phrases, she repeatedly attempted to assure me that she was not a bad mother. My attempts at gentle reassurance seemed to have only a minimal effect on her anxiety—anxiety that overwhelmed her, causing her to lose her train of thought every few minutes. This caused her great embarrassment, yet her apologies seemed only to make her more anxious. Never in her wildest dreams, she told me, would she have imagined herself speaking to a counselor!

No one had ever known her. To her acquaintances and coworkers she was the lighthearted clown who could inject humor into many situations, often making herself the butt of a self-denigrating joke.

Yet, as I was to discover, she had a private self with private symptoms. She suffered from periods of both debilitating depression and terrible anxiety. For some years, under the supervision of her internist, she had been taking an antidepressant medication for "nerves" and found it helpful. Although she always managed to function at work, frequently she felt unable to go anywhere there were people and she would spend long periods of time lying in bed in a darkened room. In time she would inform me of her fitful sleep and terrible nightmares: ghoulish nightmares of blood, violence, and murder and of killings involving almost everyone in her immediate family.

Given this situation, it was clear that we could not meaningfully discuss the problems of Sue's daughter without simultaneously attending to her own anxieties. And why this degree of anxiety? But, of course, the answer to this question would simply have to wait. Someone as frightened as Sue would have to be approached gently and carefully.

Sometimes I wonder what I would have reported to a third party had she been in one of the managed-care groups that required preauthorization for treatment. How many would have accepted my true assessment? I was working with what appeared to be a fragile, terribly anxious person who, while not without strengths, was someone with whom I needed to take whatever time necessary to establish an alliance.

What if after a first session or two I had been asked to spell out goals in behavioral terms? Would I have been clever enough to say something true, yet acceptable? And what if I said that my reading of the situation suggested that if an alliance was formed, a big "if" at the time, my sense was that treatment may very well involve years of work? What then? Fortunately, those were not issues I needed to address.

Over the ensuing weeks, Sue's anxiety lessened, we chatted more easily, and I was able to get a better sense of the overall situation in her household. Sue felt caught in the middle between her mother, who she felt manipulated her by playing on her guilt, and her troubled daughter, whose relentless sarcasm inflicted pain on everyone in the household. Sue felt she was an utter failure as daughter and mother and was unaware of any feelings of resentment toward her family.

Early on, I raised the issue with Sue that regardless of what might be troubling her daughter, she had her own share of troubles, and I indicated my willingness to talk with her about them. She did not warm to the idea.

"You're not strong enough," she said. "Neither am I. I look at things different than anyone. I'll be a pain, hard to know. What's important to me is different than others. I have no dealings with anyone." Soon after, she told me she thought she could be divided into three parts: (1) a clown, (2) someone struggling for self-respect, and (3) someone who is crying and dying.

Six months into treatment Sue revealed that throughout her childhood, since the age of two, she had been sexually abused by her alcoholic father. She related a terrible incident when, at age nine, her father called her elementary school to ask that she be sent home ostensibly to provide care for her ill mother. She arrived home to find only her father, drunk as usual, who took this opportunity to beat and rape her.

During the following years of therapy, Sue began to talk about her early memories. Gradually, there emerged a terrible story of a child who, until mid-adolescence, was routinely beaten, invaded, and humiliated at the hands of a psychopathic father, while an ineffectual mother stood passively by. Each new memory seemed worse than the preceding one and was accompanied by floods of affect which, until then, had been frozen for decades. Sue angrily told me, "The only positive thing I remember my father saying about me was that I was a good cocksucker."

Sue had a rocky time those first few years, as did our treatment relationship. She began to consider her upbringing and its consequences. "I used to think it was just the way things were," she said. "Now it seems so unfair. Not living, just existing, surviving. Never thought about how it affected me. I just *said* it affected me." Memories evoked grizzly flashbacks involving all her senses. Flashbacks of noxious odors induced marked sleeplessness and severe agitation.

And then came the full brunt of her depression, which in spite of medication increases and changes seemed untouchable. She refused hospitalization and, not unlike her worst pretreatment periods of stress, her life narrowed to work, bedrest, and therapy appointments.

My weekly appointment hour with her, which was typically supplemented with a call or two, was far and away the most demanding hour of my week. Most of my interventions fell flat, and the key thrust of my therapeutic efforts was aimed at repeatedly telling her, trying to convince myself at the same time, that there was a light at the end of the tunnel, that her depression would not go on forever, and that I would hang in there with her.

Finally things did get better. For most of the next year her mood was considerably brighter and her self-esteem much improved. To her family's dismay, she began asserting herself and setting limits on their manipulations.

She began attending weekly outings at a neighborhood restaurant with friends she had made at work. She became involved in crafts and began receiving recognition awards at local craft shows. Coworkers were delighted to see her return to better spirits, and her employer gave her increased responsibilities in a new project.

But this newfound emotional health was still too fragile to withstand the blow that was to come. Lisa, of whom Sue was especially fond, was the older daughter of Sue's former neighbor. Lisa, a young woman then in her twenties, revealed to Sue that on several occasions she too had been sexually abused by her own father during her adolescence and at times by her mother as well.

Sue became overcome with rage. The powerful identification she had with Lisa's trauma left her feeling that if she were anywhere near Lisa's parents she would kill them. She was unable to sleep for days. Reluctantly she agreed to be admitted to the hospital for what was to be the first of several brief hospital stays.

While in the hospital her flashbacks and night terrors became more severe. She began remembering in even more detail scenes of unimaginable degradation and her father's threats that he would gut her like a fish or cut off her hands if she dared tell anyone. With the help of a treatment team and a devoted social work intern, she began to talk and write about her experiences and began avidly reading accounts of other trauma victims. She attended art therapy sessions and drew pictures of her memories, including one of a giant headless man with a grotesque erect penis. The man towers over a small naked girl who cries from a face with no eyes. Within weeks Sue left the hospital remarkably stronger.

This is where an author is tempted to end a case report. I wish I could say that she lived happily ever after. But sometimes, in spite of our good work and our patients' best efforts, things do not go as we would wish.

Sometime the following year, during a family get-together, an argument became heated and a family member lost control and physically assaulted Sue. Once more she was briefly hospitalized, and once more the flashbacks and depressive symptoms returned.

Now, seven years since the start of therapy, I have grown accustomed to the fact that Sue will probably always be vulnerable to such setbacks. During the difficult times she tells me that she has no hope, that she wants to give up, and she insists that I should give up too. She tells me of her nightmares and haunting memories and her burdens of rage, guilt, and self-loathing.

I tell her that I will carry the hope until she feels stronger, and that I am not yet ready to throw in the towel. I extend myself a bit more during these times. Sometimes, at her request, we go outside and walk during our sessions and, when necessary, we arrange additional brief phone contacts through the week. Sue receives additional support and hope from the social work intern who has remained in contact with her, and from her psychiatrist, a devoted health care provider who closely monitors her medication. For the worst times, hospitalization remains an option.

I do not anticipate a change in the treatment plan in the foreseeable future.

Discussion

In my attempt to defend and justify long-term treatment, I could have presented a different kind of case for this article. I could have presented clinical material of someone healthier, of someone, for instance, who credited intensive clinical work with making a fundamental change in his or her life. I could have described someone, for instance, who claimed long-term treatment enabled him or her to save a failing marriage or to leave a hopeless one, to complete an education or change a dead-end career, to get over a developmental hurdle, or to stop the repetition of destructive patterns. There is no shortage of this type of clinical material. We have worked with many such individuals. Indeed, many of us count ourselves among them. A more successful case might have more generously supported the effectiveness of long-term treatment. After all, Sue is not a typical client. Yet I chose this case because, although it is not typical, it is not altogether rare.

I present this material to support those of us who work in clinical settings and can bear witness to the steady stream of individuals who come seeking help and whose developmental histories, although perhaps not as severe as Sue's, are nonetheless riddled with abuse, neglect, and deprivation. It seems their numbers are growing.

And many of us continue to hold fast to the belief that the ideal treatment for people who have been failed by human relationships is an enduring human relationship that does not fail. In the words of Winnicott (1987),

> In a particular way we can actually alter the patient's past, so that a patient whose maternal environment was not good enough can change into a person who has had a good-enough facilitating environment, and whose personal growth has therefore been able to take place, though late. (p. 102)

Conclusion

Winnicott stressed that mothers who have it in them to provide good-enough care can be enabled to do better by being cared for themselves in a way that acknowledges the essential nature of their task. Therapists have similar needs. Like the mothers of decades past, it becomes increasingly difficult for clinicians to trust their own good instincts when their professional institutions, colleagues, and supervisors declare that their devotion to long-term work with a suffering person is theoretically suspect or antiquated.

It is all the more difficult to lose this support when the third parties on whom we have—for better or worse—grown to rely for our living become withholding and punitive. Insurance companies that limit sessions to 12 per year, that insist on all-too-frequent case reports and case reviews, influence therapists to mistrust their skills and training and to adopt the insurance point of view in place of their own.

It is a battle for the mind of the therapist, in what Kramer (1990) referred to as the "sentinel effect." If all goes well in the insurance world, therapists will internalize a hostile sentinel and become suspicious of their own good intentions. The internalized sentinel of the insurance company fans the flames of the therapist's doubts and uncertainty. A subliminal shift will occur in the mind of the therapist. The limits of treatment covered by an insurance company will gradually be registered in the mind of the therapist as, "This is all the patient needs."

It is frightening to see where we are allowing ourselves to be led. Kramer (1990) posed the question, "If sentinel effects and restrictions on care cause us to alter our thoughts and behavior—to starve our patients and then see their hunger pangs as whining—how will we act when these pressures are universal?" (p. 23).

What we will see is a naturalistic study of parallel process. As we clinicians feel supported, as we feel held, we could, in kind, support and hold our clientele. As we feel mistrusted, hurried, and pressured, so too will this be transmitted to the people under our care and to our trainees.

In *Future Shock*, Toffler (1970) acknowledged that change is essential but warned that change unguided and unrestrained can overwhelm our defenses and erode our decision-making processes. It is this sort of runaway change, I believe, that is occurring in the mental health practices of our day. "The limits of treatment covered by an insurance company will gradually be registered in the mind of the therapist as, 'This is all the patient needs'."

Increasingly, our clinical sensibilities are being molded by the whims and pressures of the marketplace. And the pressures mount. Today's clinician, interviewed as a prospective provider for an insurance company, is subjected to managed-care McCarthyism. But it is not communism that must be disavowed, but beliefs in a long-term treatment relationship, even though we know, particularly because of our heritage as clinical social workers, that a reliable, enduring relationship is no less necessary for the tormented individual of today than it was for such individuals in days gone by.

We, and especially the next generation of clinicians, stand to lose the clinical wisdom that has been painstakingly accumulated, refined, and passed down from our teachers and supervisors. We must work to ensure that the legacy of this knowledge continues to be transmitted to our students and supervisees.

And finally, we clinicians must maintain and strengthen our connections with each other, individually and through our professional organizations, so that, especially in harried times like these—when so much of the health care world seems pressured, confusing, and reckless—we can find for ourselves, among kindred spirits, a holding environment.

Note

1 This chapter first published as Meyer, W. S. (1993). In defense of long-term treatment: On the vanishing holding environment. *Social Work, 38*(5), 571–578. Copyright © 1993. Reprinted by permission of Oxford University Press. An earlier version of the article was presented at the National Federation of Societies for Clinical Social Work's 20th Anniversary Clinical Conference, September 1991, Boston, and at the North Carolina Society for Clinical Social Work, March 1992, Durham, NC. Accepted February 26, 1992.

References

Boardroom Classics. (Ed.). (1989). *The book of inside information*. New York: Board Room Reports.

Castelnuovo-Tedesco, P. (1971). Decreasing the length of psychotherapy: Theoretical and practical aspects of the problem. In S. Arieti (Ed.), *The world biennial of psychiatry and psychotherapy* (pp. 55–71). New York: Basic Books.

Castelnuovo-Tedesco, P. (1990). [Letter to the editor]. *American Journal of Psychiatry, 147*, 1258.

DeAngelis, T. (1989, July). Personal events pave road to understanding. *Monitor*, p. 38.

Good, P. R. (1987). Brief therapy in the age of Reagapeutics. *American Journal of Orthopsychiatry, 57*, 6–11.

Halpert, E. (1972). The effect of insurance on psychoanalytic treatment. *Journal of the American Psychoanalytic Association, 20*, 122–133.

Halpert, E. (1973). A meaning of insurance in psychotherapy. *International Journal of Psychoanalytic Psychotherapy, 1*, 62–68.

Kanter, J. (1990). Community-based management of psychotic clients. *Clinical Social Work Journal, 18*, 23–42.

Kramer, P. D. (1990, November). Dino or dodo? *Psychiatric Times*, p. 23.

Mackenzie, K. R. (1991). Principles of brief intensive psychotherapy. *Psychiatric Annals, 21*, 398–404.

Michaels, E. (1989). BPP: Psychotherapy that takes weeks, not years. *Canadian Medical Association Journal, 140*, 842–843.

Modell, A. (1976). "The holding environment" and the therapeutic action of psychoanalysis. *Journal of the American Psychoanalytic Association, 24*, 285–308.

Rodman, F. R. (1987). *The spontaneous gesture: Selected letters of D. W. Winnicott*. Cambridge, MA: Harvard University Press.

Stone, L. (1954). The widening scope of indications for psychoanalysis. *Journal of the American Psychoanalytic Association, 2*, 567–594.

Toffler, A. (1970). *Future shock*. New York: Random House.

Winnicott, D. W. (1965). *The maturational process and the facilitating environment*. New York: International Universities Press.

Winnicott, D. W. (1987). *Babies and their mothers.* Reading, PA: Addison-Wesley.
Wolfenstein, M. (1953). Trends in infant care. *American Journal of Orthopsychiatry, 23*, 120–130.
Zuckerman, R. L. (1989). Iatrogenic factors in "managed" psychotherapy. *American Journal of Psychotherapy, 63*, 118–131.

Chapter 5

Long-term treatment in the rearview mirror

William S. Meyer

It is intriguing for me to reread my paper, "In Defense of Long-Term Treatment" now 26 years old, which included my assessment and interactions with Sue, some seven years into our work together. I suggested in the article that treatment was likely to continue for an indeterminate period. I could not have been more prescient, in that our work together was to continue for a total of 30 years. While Sue generally did what she could to put on her best game face – and when she was on, she had a terrific sense of humor – there were stretches when Sue suffered from unremitting depression and deep feelings of hopelessness.

I will soon return to discussing my work with Sue, even though she was not the primary inspiration for me to write that paper. While I make no mention of it in the article, what prompted me, at that time, to write defending long-term treatment was a suicidal crisis involving a patient of mine, John, a depressed, Duke college freshman. My experience with John was too fresh and too raw to write about at the time and I was too emotionally vulnerable to expose myself.

John

I don't remember much about John, a depressed college freshman at Duke, first time away from home, because his time in treatment with me was so brief. What I do remember is that it was during a time when managed care was pervading the mental health field and all practitioners could feel its presence. There it was, lurking over our shoulders, assessing every diagnosis, every treatment decision, every clinical appointment, and every treatment plan.

It was not that I was unsympathetic to why managed care entered the mental health marketplace. I had worked on inpatient psychiatric units and knew that abuse of the system was common. I had seen long-term hospitalizations provided for people who could have done just as well in outpatient treatment – adults with chronic personality disturbances and teenagers whose problems were no more serious than getting caught smoking marijuana – hospitalized for weeks and months at a time, provided the patients had multi-million-dollar mental health insurance policies. As a consequence, there was a proliferation of newly built private psychiatric hospitals, which served little purpose other than to drain such funds from insurance companies. A common scenario: Patients would be kept in the hospital because they were deemed too ill for discharge. When their insurance ran out, however, and they could no longer remain in private institutional care, the patients would be transferred to the local state hospital which provided care for the most ill patients in much less plush surroundings than private hospitals could provide. Miraculously, most of these patients, within weeks, days, or even hours, were suddenly well enough to go home, and they and their families would be clamoring for immediate discharge.

When hospitals were monetarily incentivized to keep patients as long as possible, *managed care was necessary* to provide oversight to determine when longer-term psychiatric hospitalizations were medically necessary. Unfortunately, this oversight became overarching in all aspects of mental health care, even outpatient care, in all psychiatric clinics, including our own at Duke. The expectation of working quickly and briefly and the frenetic atmosphere it created was becoming pervasive in psychiatry departments and mental health clinics throughout the US. The message was clear: treatments were to be short-term – the quicker, the better. As I mentioned in the original article, managed care was having a "sentinel effect." It was a battle for the mind of the therapist, in which therapists would internalize a hostile sentinel guarding against and thwarting any inclination toward longer-term treatments.

The effect this had on clinicians was profound, and the needs of the patient were replaced by whatever the insurance covered. Clinicians, especially those newer to the field, were inclined to mistrust themselves and trust the communications from the insurance companies. Clinical training in every mental health profession was altered to promote brief treatments. Frequently, programs justified this type of training by saying "we need to prepare the clinician of tomorrow by teaching them the clinical skills that insurance companies will pay for." It cannot be overstated how thoroughly and long-lasting an influence this had on clinical thinking.

With John, I felt pressure to hurry my assessment, rush my treatment, accompanied by the pressure to bring treatment to its quickest possible conclusion. Managed care was omnipresent in our clinic and it affected everything I was doing, not only with John, but with everyone I was seeing at the time. Prior to that time, I was told by supervisors to slow down, take my time, get to know the patient, not to rush to judgment either about diagnosis or treatment.

After the very few sessions that John and I met, during which time I was hurriedly trying to get him to be less symptomatic, I received a call from an administrative dean informing me that John had slit his wrists and would be taking medical leave from the school. Perhaps only a practicing psychotherapist can fully imagine how devastating it is to receive such a call. I was horrified and guilt-ridden, convinced that my departure from my usual, gradual way of getting to know a new patient contributed substantively to this sad outcome.

Long term treatment? For whom?

In my original article, I used the clinical example of my seven years of work with Sue, not anticipating that my work with her would last so long. I had chosen the case because she had suffered childhood abuse in the extreme, and my rationale was that no one would argue against long-term care for someone who had been subjected to such severe maltreatment. At the time, I thought it necessary to use such an extreme case to bolster my argument that people who had such horrific backgrounds, often required long periods of time in treatment. What I didn't appreciate at the time, due to my relative inexperience, was just how varied are the patients who need or are helped by long-term care.

To be clear, not everyone I see wants or needs long-term therapy. In my practice, some people want to be seen only a few sessions, some for months, others for years, and still others indeterminately. After formal therapy concludes, some stay in touch with me via e-mail and others still may wish to come in on occasion. Moreover, at one time it was assumed that a geographical move on the part of the patient or therapist automatically ended the therapy. Now, with the increased use of video conferencing, this opens an opportunity for therapeutic work to continue long-distance.

Dr. S.

Dr. S., a prominent physician, who is gay, entered therapy when he was in his thirties. Although his parents, both physicians, cared for him, his life became bleak when, at age six, he was sent for 18 months to a boarding school. The school was run by a sadistic headmaster. Beatings were commonplace and bullying and cruelty by the other boys was an everyday occurrence.

Although he had long considered himself to be his mother's favorite, when at the age of 18 he came out to her, she said, "You are an abomination. I wish you had never been born." At the age of 28 he fell in love with a male roommate and enjoyed a deep friendship that was intimate, but not sexual. When Dr. S. ultimately confessed to his roommate his more amorous feelings, the roommate hastily moved out.

Dr. S. felt lonely and rejected and turned to drugs to compensate. For the next four years he was hooked on amphetamines. By the time he was 32, he was taking huge doses every day, and at night, chloral hydrate, a hypnotic, to sleep. He began calling in sick at work, sometimes for days at a time, and lost nearly 80 pounds in three months. Nearly one year later, almost always under the influence of some substance, he presented himself for treatment to a male psychiatrist/psychoanalyst, who was approximately his same age. He wrote of that experience,

> I was suspicious ... he was so young ... What experience of life, what therapeutic power, I thought could I find in someone scarcely older than myself? I soon realized that this was someone of exceptional character ... someone who felt I could tolerate and profit from intensive analysis ...

But the psychiatrist insisted that for treatment to continue, Dr. S. must give up drugs, whose use, he said, made success in treatment impossible. Dr. S. never took amphetamines again and wrote that treatment had saved his life many times over. Neither he nor his friends thought he would make it past his mid-thirties. Dr. S. saw his psychiatrist twice a week for nearly five decades!

While the psychiatrist, Leonard Shengold, is known mostly in psychoanalytic circles, particularly for his work and books on "Soul Murder" (1989, 1999), the patient is the beloved, world-renowned author and neurologist, the late Oliver Sacks. The story above is detailed in two books in particular, (Sacks, 2001, 2015); the second memoir, written when Sacks was past 80.

Of note, shortly after Sacks' 75th birthday he met a man named "Billy." To quote Sacks, "Timid and inhibited all my life, I let a friendship and intimacy grow between us ..." Shortly thereafter, Billy told Sacks, "I have conceived a deep love for you." Sacks writes,

> I had conceived a deep love for him too – and my eyes filled with tears ... It was a new experience for me to lie quietly in someone's arms and talk, or listen to music, or be silent together ... We have a tranquil, many-dimensional sharing of our lives – a great and unexpected gift in my old age, after a lifetime of keeping at a distance.

Who can say which persons can benefit from long-term treatment and how long such treatment should take?

Long-term treatment or brief? If an individual was on a psychotropic medicine that provided symptom relief, would anyone suggest that the person stop taking it? If anything, patients are generally discouraged, and usually strongly so, from tampering with a drug regimen that has demonstrated efficacy. How ironic then, that if it is a human relationship that helps someone feel better, most individuals who have influence in the mental health field (supervisors, insurance companies, mental health agencies) press to know when the date for will be for, of all words, *termination*. Victor Bloom (1997) remarked that he had a patient say, "I don't want to get well; if I did, I wouldn't be able to see you anymore." In reality, Bloom notes, the therapy was the most gratifying situation in the patient's life. For the patient, it was worth every penny, because in the session, the therapist's attention, ameliorating the patient's yearning to be loved and understood, was being gratified, albeit not completely. Why should a patient fear that getting well will necessarily result in the loss of a therapist? As Bergmann (1997) has noted, for many patients, the therapeutic relationship is the best love relationship they have ever experienced.

Sue

While nearly all of my clinical work is standard psychotherapy, built on the convention of the 50-minute, office-based hour, I have always allowed for an unconventional approach to therapy, tailoring what I do to the unique needs of any individual patient. Sue was very special to me. I had been impacted not only by the severity and chronicity of the many traumas in her life, but how, despite such suffering, she maintained her perseverance, dignity, and warm humor. Our work together evolved into a deep, mutually rewarding and intimate collaboration that was anything but conventional.

How unconventional? In the early work of our treatment, Sue found meeting in my hospital-based office too confining, and we had our sessions strolling through the hospital grounds. Sue was a chronic smoker, and once, I told her I would take her to a local baseball game of the famous Durham Bulls, if she would even consider stopping smoking. She knew I would not in any way shame her for trying and that my offer was one of caring for her well-being. We went to the ball game, and while the smoking abated for a time, she resumed within weeks. I took her out to lunch once a year for her birthday and accompanied her to her first visit to a senior citizen's center in the hopes of helping her be more social. Despite this unconventional approach, I took care that no professional ethical boundary would ever be crossed.

Throughout my career within Duke's Department of Psychiatry I have been involved in training psychiatric residents. Once each year, I would arrange for Sue to give a lecture to them about what it is that helps patients. She would use her clinical relationship with me as a case example. Her favorite admonition was to remind them that they should never talk to patients like they were "reading from a textbook," a trait of mine that she brought up with me with some frequency during the early years of our work. Many psychiatry trainees told me how meaningful their interchange with Sue was, and I know that for her it was an annual event that brought her great joy, as she, with only a high school diploma, was "teaching" the psychiatrists of the future.

Sue's final days

When I met Sue, she was still residing with her mother, having never lived on her own. Ultimately, I worked with Sue for over three decades, seeing her in our early years through several psychiatric hospitalizations, through the death of her mother with whom she lived, then through several moves.

While our counseling sessions allowed Sue the opportunity to tell her story, our most important therapeutic goal was for Sue to get to know how she truly felt and to enable true self-expression with those around her. Although the majority of our time was spent in my listening to and providing psychotherapy for Sue, I, as perhaps only a clinical social worker would, provided concrete help in many ways as well. I supported and helped her through several relocations, from an apartment to a trailer, then to housing for the disabled. Later, when she developed crippling medical problems, I helped her move to a nursing home, where I visited her intermittently. While I did not participate in the actual moves themselves, I arranged for someone to deliver some used furniture from my family to hers and I was able to procure for her a computer from which through e-mail she would update me about her personal life. Usually, however, she would simply send me cartoons and witty postings that she found amusing. I wanted very much for her to have as full a life as possible and did whatever I could to encourage her in that direction, while also providing some of that fullness when I could.

Once, in an e-mail, she wrote me this:

Any time I am with you I feel like a weight has been taken off me. I get to smile and laugh with you. There is so much beauty in this world. Sometimes it falls in your lap, other times you have to look hard to see it. Just thank you again for everything you had given me, for my mind and for fun. A song that is in my top 5 is "winter summer or fall, you will be there when I call." Every word is what you mean to me and so much more. All I can work on now is getting well at this time.

It has been near 30 years. I am so happy we are still friends. My heart just feels so warm when I think about you, and your caring for me. You have such a big heart, thank you for putting up with me during all that has gone on in my life for so long.

I will never forget one thing.

Always your friend, Sue

Much of our treatment involved helping her with life's challenges and helping her to remain out of the hospital, which she succeeded in doing for at least the last 25 years of our collaborative work. She knew how hard I tried for her and the depth of my sympathy for all that she had been through in this life. The type of work I'd done with her contained elements of "supportive psychotherapy" (Werman, 1984), case management (Kanter, 2000) and even palliative psychotherapy. In a brief essay on the latter topic, Kahn (2011) wrote that it is therapy whose goal it is to make another's existence "a little less lonely and painful."

A couple of years ago, I got a call from one of Sue's relatives, informing me that Sue had suffered a severe stroke, had been rushed to a nearby hospital, and was lying comatose. The call came during a weekend and I was able to make it to the hospital and plant a kiss on my dear friend's cheek, the day before she died.

To illustrate one small element of our work, there came a time when we focused primarily on the need for her to stand up for herself to family and friends. I tapped into her sense of humor at the end of one session by saying, "Now this week, don't take no shit off nobody." Sue loved that line and for years we would say this to each other at the end of every session. During this period, she told me about a television program she had just seen. I was so moved that I wrote a poem about it and gave it to her as a holiday gift. In the poem, I mention a patient encounter I had in the high-risk obstetrics clinic, where, in addition to my psychotherapy practice, I have now worked for the past 20 years.

She had the poem framed and kept it at her bedside:

FOR SUE,
AND THE VANQUISHED SOULS OF BABY ELEPHANTS

"I just saw a TV show about an elephant," you told me.
"I used to be just like him.
When he was a baby they chained his ankle.
He squealed and squirmed until there was no more fight left in him.
He was just too puny to pull away.
Now he has a chain around his mind.
His baby memories run so deep he doesn't realize that now he is grown and powerful.
Why he could pull that chain out of the ground any old time he wants to.
He just doesn't know it. So all he does is stand there.
I used to be just like him."

I remembered how our weeks of therapy turned into months turned into years.
You couldn't trust me at first. No wonder, given the nightmare that was your childhood.
Over time, our therapy became infused with love.
You brought me your pain, your courage, your integrity, your warmth, and your humor.
Once at the end of a session I looked you square-in-the-eye and said, "Now this week, don't take no shit off nobody!" You laughed.
At the end of the next session, you looked me square-in-the-eye and said, "Now don't you take no shit off nobody!" We both laughed.
And so it went. Every week we would end the session with a square-in-the-eye-look and say, "Now don't take no shit off nobody!"

It was a good way to end our sessions.
Link by link your long chain fell away.

Yesterday, in clinic, I saw a wisp of a woman who had a pregnant belly and a blackened eye.
She had come to her appointment with HIM.
HE had dark glasses and stank of alcohol.
"I bumped my head on a door," she lied to me.
I looked through her medical chart. An emergency room visit, and Another, and ANOTHER.
she had been hit, Punched, PUSHed and KICKED.
I dug back through her chart to when she was a child.
abuse, abUSE, ABUSE. bad parents, Foster Care, MORE FOSTER CARE.
"I can help you," I told her.
"I can get you in a shelter that will keep you safe. Just don't leave here with HIM."
HE had already started down the hallway. HE looked back with a dagger-eyed glare.
First at me, then at her.
What HE expected was clear.
She walked – toward HIM, paused, turned around and – for one eternal moment – fixed her eyes upon mine.
I pleaded with my look. As hard as I possibly could.
But she lifted her chin, did a half-pirouette, and flashed her sad smile – at HIM.
Arms entangled, they departed.
All I could do was stand there. And watch them get smaller in the distance.

Perhaps one day, like you, she will find the land where the elephants all run free.

References

Bergmann, M.S. (1997). Termination: The Achilles heel of psychoanalytic technique. *Psychoanalytic Psychology*, *14*, 163–174.

Bloom, V. (1997). Interminable analysis? *Journal of the American Academy of Psychoanalysis and Dynamic Psychaitry*, *25*(2), 313–316.

Kahn, M.W. (2011). Palliative psychotherapy. *American Journal of Psychiatry*, *168*(9), 888–889.

Kanter, J. (2000). Beyond psychotherapy: Therapeutic relationships in community care. *Smith College Studies in Social Work*, *70*(3), 397–426.

Sacks, O. (2001). *Uncle Tungsten: Memories of a chemical boyhood.* New York, NY: Vintage Books.

Sacks, O. (2015). *On the move: A life.* New York, NY: Alfred A. Knopf.

Shengold, L. (1989). *Soul murder: The effects of childhood abuse and deprivation.* New York, NY: Ballantine Books.

Shengold, L. (1999). *Soul murder revisited: Thoughts about therapy, hate, love and memory.* New Haven, CT: Yale University Press.

Werman, D.S. (1984). *The practice of supportive psychotherapy.* New York, NY: Brunner/Mazel.

Part II

Trauma and issues of attachment

Chapter 6

Mourning the melancholy object

Giving voice to traumatic experience

Carol Ganzer

What has captured my attention in reading recent literature (Frosh, 2013; Grand & Salberg, 2017; Harris, Kalb, & Klebanoff, 2016; Salberg & Grand, 2017) about psychoanalytically oriented treatment is writing that investigates how patients, as well as therapists, are haunted by early trauma, unresolved mourning, and unconscious, dissociated, or unformulated thoughts. As a result, they live out their experiences in the consulting room through projections and enactments. In working with traumatic experience, I believe it is necessary for treatment to extend over the course of many years for enough trust to be established, for roles to be enacted, to recognize what was possibly carried from our histories into the therapeutic space in mourned and unmourned losses.

Long-term treatment with an individual tends to deepen the relationship, allowing the patient to internalize me as a good object, manage traumatic triggers, exhibit growth in personal relationships, recognize old patterns of behavior and have a deeper and more expansive lived experience. The benefits of these relationships also accrue to me as well. In short, therapist and patient are less haunted by their early experience, able to resolve therapeutic impasses, and open space for mutual recognition when they engage in long-term treatment.

In this chapter I will discuss clinical encounters from a ten-year treatment of a woman whose protracted mourning of her father made it difficult to be emotionally available to others or to allow others to be available to her. The absent father, coupled with a harsh, critical, and often inattentive mother, were roles that were enacted in the therapeutic relationship creating impasses in the treatment and a feeling of emptiness in the patient and frustration in me. A statement by the patient about how her father's death affected her led to my disclosure of a similar traumatic experience in my history. Subsequently, my reverie and reflection on an unformulated or forgotten experience of my own enabled me to shift my position in the treatment and metabolize both my feelings and the patient's. This clinical moment resulted in opening space for us to begin a process where she could use me as a good object. She, in turn, began to complete her mourning process. I recognized that I too had been haunted and lived out an unmourned relationship with my father. I investigate what ghosts haunt us, either acknowledged or unacknowledged, how they thwart our work, how they enter the treatment through absence and silence, and what might be censored and unsayable by both parties. In the end, I reflect on what broke through the impasses and enabled both patient and therapist to speak.

Much of what we do in therapeutic work is to deal with ghosts from the past and haunting that lies hidden, often unrecognized, interfering with the grieving process and with freeing ourselves from the loss of the loved object. According to Frosh (2013), the melancholy object is "one that is never fully acknowledged and consequently can never be properly mourned, which means that it is somehow preserved in a kind of half-life" (p. 39). Further, Frosh argues, "it is not only the object that is both lost and preserved, it is also awareness of that object" (p. 39). It is a "present absence" that invades, casting a dark shadow over the individual (p. 121). It is this object that makes its appearance in the following treatment.

Case illustration

Harper initially contacted me because she believed that she became involved with "unavailable men" and despaired of ever meeting anyone with whom she might have a serious commitment. The colleague who referred Harper to me thought she needed to work on her relationship with her mother, and a significant portion of our early work involved exploring what transpired between her mother and her. During the first three years of our work together we met weekly. Her father had died when she was aged 25 after a lifelong battle with diabetes. Her mother and older sister were very close and lived in proximity to each other. In the early years of treatment, Harper spoke of the difficulties she had in establishing relationships. I thought perhaps her feelings that others were not available to her stemmed from her relationship with her mother, who never seemed emotionally available but nonetheless was highly critical; they often engaged in verbal battles.

Harper had shared numerous examples of her mother's behavior, shifting from intrusiveness to total neglect. Harper's mother encouraged her to have bariatric surgery at age 28 due to a history of diabetes and hypertension in the family. Reluctantly, Harper complied, but when her mother suggested she have a breast reduction as well, she refused to schedule the surgery. When Harper's sister had a destination wedding in Jamaica, Harper was not included in the plans, but not only did they invite a neighbor who had previously dated her mother, they also covered his accommodations and airfare. After her father died, Harper's mother left her alone in the house and moved in with her older sister for a period of time. "She totally shut me out, not being a mother," Harper lamented. "She said 'I can't be around you, it's so depressing.'"

Harper's father had died of serious complications from diabetes several years before she began treatment with me. She described their relationship as very close. They shared a sense of humor, liberal political views, and a commitment to social justice issues. She was distraught after his death and engaged in treatment with a male therapist for about a year. I learned over time that she often wore her father's wedding ring and was very devoted to his memory, continuing to mourn the loss. When I learned about the origin of the ring, I asked about its significance. She indicated it was the only piece of jewelry she had, and she liked wearing it. She remarked in a session that when she had talked about her father with a young man she was dating, he thought her father was still alive by the way she described him. I then began to realize that in a sense time had stopped with her father's death. "Every day," she said, "I relive it. I still remember the morning, still hear his voice, still smell the hospital room, what he looked like after he died." Slowly, it became clear that the feeling that men were unavailable to her may have had more to do with her father's absence than her mother's neglect, and that she was repeating her traumatic loss with each attempt to form a relationship. Symbolically she was married to her father, and his ghostlike spectre claimed her allegiance.

I started to pay more attention to the ways in which Harper engaged in her relationships with the men she met. When she finally did find a relationship, and was engaged to be married, the relationship fell apart after they moved in together and he became controlling, physically and verbally abusive, and tried to choke her. I worried that I had missed something in our work that was now being acted out in her relationship. Her transference to me had been fairly positive over the several years we had worked together, but I felt that she kept much of her emotional life hidden from me.

The shift in treatment

After the last altercation with her fiancé, Harper ended their relationship, and we began more frequent contact, moving from weekly to three times a week contact. I was not prepared for what ensued. Harper arrived for her first few sessions wearing pajamas. They looked like children's pajamas, with a teddy bear figure printed on the fabric. What, I asked myself is she showing me? The sessions took place in my home office late in the evening. Pajamas? Does she want to be tucked in? Does she have fantasies of moving into my home? I asked about the pajamas. Her response was that it was late; she would be going home after the session and was prepared for bed.

Shortly after we increased the frequency of our sessions, I sent Harper a short video about psychoanalysis that I found on the internet. She responded by sending me a video called, "The Honey Badger," that portrayed an aggressive wild animal devouring its prey. The honey badger survived and appeared impervious to the attacks. I pursued the meaning of this video with Harper because she sent it in response to my offer of a deeper treatment. I wondered aloud if she feared being devoured by the process or had an aggressive wish to devour me. Rather nonchalantly, she replied that either was possible, "Isn't the therapist sometimes *the rapist*?" splitting the word in two. She then showed me a cartoon on her iPhone that depicted a therapist's door with those two words, THE RAPIST, in bold letters. I felt uneasy and uncertain as to how to proceed.

Although Harper eagerly increased the sessions, and used the couch immediately, she began having difficulty finding words to speak about her experiences and feelings. She often felt frustrated and thought that she had nothing to say in session, a change from our weekly psychotherapy sessions. It seemed to me that the silences were enactments of something in her history, possibly emerging from the increased frequency of our sessions. At first, I thought I was experiencing what it was like for Harper to be with her mother, who was distracted, forgetful, and emotionally unavailable.

Although Harper brought a few dreams to her treatment, they were either scenes of rescuing me or invading my home. In one dream she brought she was breaking into my house or found herself there and wanted to get out. I asked her what she thought it might mean that she was there without my knowledge. "I didn't want to scare you," she responded. I queried, "Do you think you might scare me?" She did not reply to my question, and when I tried to explore what might be scary about seeing her, she changed the subject to wanting another tattoo. I brought up the video she sent me about the honey badger devouring its prey and wondered if she viewed breaking and entering my home in the dream as an aggressive action. I thought about the interactions she had with her mother that disintegrated into bitter accusations and name-calling and wondered if she was possibly setting the stage for similar interactions with me and feared them. The dream suggested an ambivalent position, breaking and entering and wanting to get out.

After this dream she talked less and less in each session. She was restless on the couch, moving about, shifting her arms and legs, unable to settle herself. She asked to shorten the sessions from 50 to 45 minutes, she pled with me to leave early. She often canceled and rescheduled her session. I found myself meeting with her at odd times, on Sunday, late at night, by phone. She had little to say, a few snippets of conversation. I attempted to interpret the silences as communication, that she was saying something without words and showing me through her actions, not telling me. What could she not say?

The shift in the therapist

I began to experience the sessions as long and tedious, wishing I had not agreed to increased sessions. I felt trapped, controlled, and irritated by her behavior. I knew that we were enacting something, but I was uncertain what it was. To say that Harper was resisting would be an easy way out. It let me off the hook. She was certainly provocative in her behaviors, pulling me to change times, meet on weekend hours, asking for revisions to the frame. It is possible that Harper was testing my limits and pushing me to bend the frame; and by doing so, I hoped to better understand what we were enacting. Who in her internal world was being evoked by her relationship with me? As I am fairly interactive with all of my patients, I knew that I must be paying a role in keeping her silent and contributing to the impasse in the treatment. Who was I and who was she in this particular drama? I had often thought that we were playing out maternal roles in our work, with me being the loving mother and Harper being the critic, but I found myself falling into feeling critical and impatient with her, thus playing out the role between my mother and me. She was demanding and difficult, neither wanting to stay or go, but testing me with each session as to my ability to provide what she was seeking. Instead of our increased frequency making it easier for Harper to use me as a good object, I became instead projections of a negative one. We had reached an impasse, or an entanglement around the frame, in a battle for power and control of the treatment.

In exploring clinical interaction, Harris (2009) proposed paying "attention to the analyst's internal world as participating in analytic process, to impasse and then to change and momentum" (p. 6). Also, concerning therapeutic impasses, Harris (2009) considered them as "linked to an impasse in some forms of mourning in the analyst" (p. 2). I pondered that reference, but at the time could not locate a site of mourning in myself. Davies (2004) also, conjectured that "I have come to think of certain impasses in psychoanalytic work not as enactment one can't get out of, but rather as nascent enactments one can't fully enter and get into" (p. 730). Were we in a liminal space, teetering on the edge of an enactment? If so, what part was I playing in preventing us from opening a potential space to play out our various self-states or conscious or unconscious internalized object relationships? Why, instead, had the space collapsed into relative silence?

A co-created space

It is my experience that we are enacting all the time in clinical work, whether it is a brief moment, a dramatic act, or the entirety of the treatment. I view enactment as an intersubjective process occurring between therapist and patient. No longer considered as solely a behavior by the patient, enactment involves the participation of the therapist and is co-constructed between therapist and patient. This mutual participation is a primary means of entering the internal world of the other. The patient, in repeating patterns of behaviors, together with identifications and projections from internalized object relationships, sets the stage for maintaining ties to those early objects.

While the therapist's participation in these scenarios is often unintended and/or unconscious, it is nonetheless inevitable.

In this manner, the patient and therapist live out experiences derived from their histories and inner lives in the transference/countertransference field. It is living through, recognizing, and reflecting upon these enactments that are the central means of promoting therapeutic action and change in the patient, as well as in the therapist. How do we identify and use these enactments when they seem conceptually complex and clinically intimidating? From a relational perspective, we can no longer sit comfortably outside of the treatment, holding, containing, or only interpreting. As Mitchell (1988) so aptly described, we are embedded in the process, and it is both inevitable and necessary that we enact and play roles from various self-states of both participants in the treatment. As Aron (1991) has suggested, often it is difficult to tell who began the enactment. At times it is the patient, but it could equally as well be the analyst. The manner in which we identify and work our way out of enactments is through reflecting on our thoughts and behaviors. What signals an enactment for me is a disturbance in the field. I find myself behaving differently from my usual patterns with patients, or I am surprised and caught off guard in some way. Both of these realizations occurred in my work with Harper.

I began to consider the repetitive cycle in which Harper and I were caught, my withdrawal in response to her withholding, and her silence triggering something from my own history that initially was unconscious. The ways in which Harper's mother treated her as an object resonated with me, and in the transference pulled from me intense countertransference feelings that I enacted with Harper. Tension arose around Harper's wanting to take control of the sessions by changing the schedule, meeting on the phone, leaving early, lapsing into silence, or declaring she just had nothing to say. These incidents would get under my skin. As a result, my tone of voice and body language, no doubt communicated my frustration. What blind spot in me was co-creating this discomfort and enacting it with Harper in her tendency to withdraw? Finally, I realized what irritated me about the situation. Often, I compared Harper to my other patients, who were verbally appreciative of our work and who elicited feelings of closeness from me that I did not experience with her. Harper, on the other hand, appeared to devalue my efforts by wanting to leave the sessions early, or stating she was feeling bored and listless. In an effort to explore our relationship, I disclosed the following to Harper: "I feel close to you when you tell me things, like about how you are depressed, but at other times I feel like I am chasing after you to keep you here." I was curious about what she thought about what I said.

She reluctantly responded, "It's the longest therapy I've had. Sometimes it's inconvenient, but what else can I do?" It seemed to me that my own omnipotent leanings and narcissistic investment in my work were keeping me at a distance from Harper. I tried to understand it in terms of Harper's experience of her mother who was inconsistent, stimulating but withholding, and in general unavailable. My own needs for recognition and validation, absent in my early life, were not unlike those of Harper's mother who always put her needs first. By wanting to take control of the sessions, Harper was showing me how it felt to be her in a battle to gain a sense of agency with those closest to her, a conflict that was being repeated in her romantic relationships as well. When Harper began to get close to a man, he accused her of being demanding and invasive or critical and argumentative. Harper failed to understand these criticisms, but I thought of them as aspects of her mother with which she had identified, which she then had internalized and projected onto others.

When I experienced Harper devaluing me, it seemed that Harper again identified with her inconsistent and unavailable mother, becoming the aggressor, while I was cast into Harper's position in relation to her mother who bore a resemblance to my own mother. The more I relaxed around Harper's reluctance, the less Harper made demands to push the limits. Nearing the end of one session, about a year and a half into the period of our increased sessions, I had another insight into Harper's behavior. I saw the time edging beyond 45 minutes. This moment was the first time Harper did not ask to leave early. She seemed more relaxed and engaged, and I felt another shift in our work together. Then Harper said, "Isn't it time?" I responded, "I was just going to tell you." As she got up from the couch, Harper remarked, "I'm always waiting to get cut off." I commented that it was an interesting statement and wondered if that was why she always wants to end the session, so that I am not the one doing it. She nodded affirmatively.

I then recalled that very early in our treatment Harper told me that she wished I were her mother, but when I bought this up later, she looked surprised and responded shockingly, "I said that?" disavowing her comments. How did I move from being the good, desired object to the critical, rejected one? More importantly, how would I work thorough the impasse that we created? I noted as well that her father's wedding ring was still prominently displayed on her ring finger, conjuring up ghostlike thoughts and a recent dream she had related to me where she was bringing her father to me, but he was resisting and wanting to move in another direction. When I explored the possible meaning of the dream with her, she had some thoughts about wanting her dad to know about our relationship. "You," she said, "are the most constant person in my life." When we returned several sessions later to exploring her discomfort in the sessions and her lapsing into silence, I reminded her of this earlier comment. "I am thinking of your choices of unavailable men, Harper, and with me, some part of you isn't available."

The ties to her father represented both a "familiar" and "familial" connection resulting, however, in Harper staying stuck in and being unable to complete the mourning process (Mitchell, 1988, p. 219). This tendency to preserve early connections to absent and internal objects allowed her to manage her anxiety and provided a sense of security, albeit a false one. Harper remained wed to her father because he was once available to her, and the connection preserved her sense of self. On occasion I would mention, in passing, my mothering behaviors, being available to her, rescheduling sessions, validating her experience. Rather than allow for a new object experience and a different internalized object relationship, Harper rejected my overtures for closeness and held tenaciously to the memory of her deceased father as the only good object. Meanwhile, no available men appeared on the horizon, just a string of false starts.

The self-disclosure

In a moment of frustration about two years into our increased frequency of sessions and five years into our work together, Harper exclaimed, "The wrong parent died!" She was near tears, an unusual occurrence. The comment gave me pause, as this was my story as well. My father, a remote, silent, ill, and depressed figure in my childhood, died when I was an adolescent. I rarely think about my relationship with him or how the relationship played out in my life. Most of my therapeutic work has been around the internalized relationship with my mother, her engulfment of me, her porous boundaries, her demeaning and critical commentary about my life, and the ways in which I have internalized her and acted in critical, depreciating ways with others. Even my analyst said, "You worked out your issues with your father with Dr. K." But did I? Many years after we terminated treatment, I learned that Dr. K's own father left when he was one year old, and he did not meet him again until he was 40. What might have been dissociated or even unformulated for him? What did it mean for his treatment with me and my emotionally unavailable father that his was literally absent? As I remember it, I frequently felt that Dr. K was withholding and unavailable until well into my treatment with him. These revelations led me to make a disclosure to Harper that would resonate with both of us about ghosts, mourned and unmourned.

When we reflected on Harper's experience of the wrong parent dying, I thought for a moment and then conveyed to her that this was my story as well. My father had died, and I was left with a critical and demanding mother. She said very little about my disclosure, except to affirm her own experience. What occurred next was a series of crises in Harper's life that catapulted her into a state of chaos and ultimately brought her closer to me and able to begin using me as a good object. She was terminated from her employment while her place of employment was under criminal investigation due to a co-worker's fraudulent actions. Despite having many interviews, she could not find another position. In a moment of distraction, she slammed her car into another vehicle at a red light. Finally, she learned she was pregnant by a man who had no interest in fathering a child or engaging in a committed relationship with her. She became anxious about whether or not she could continue to pay rent on her loft space or, of necessity, would need to move in with her mother.

Through this process of seeming fragmentation, Harper began to confide in me and talk about her wishes, needs, and fears. I had fantasies of moving her into the spare bedroom in my home or giving her money to pay her rent. I became more empathic to how frightened and alone she was, and I stopped harboring aggressive feelings toward her. Gradually, she began to restructure her life. Her attendance to treatment became regular and, often, I would have to end the sessions as she was talking beyond the scheduled 50 minutes. One evening as she was getting ready to leave, she turned to me and said, "I know I need you, I can say it now." What brought about this change? And what made me available to her now, when for nearly two years I had felt shut out and shut down?

Returning to where patient and therapist together inhabit negative space, Davies (2004) asserted that it is not only a moment "we have come to think of as a therapeutic impasse, but a moment of profound mutuality and engagement as well" (p. 714). We become "bad objects" for our patients "... and ... allow for the expression of their more aggressive, hateful, and malignant thoughts" (p. 714). But the challenge we face is how to "evoke the bad object relationship without concretely becoming the bad objects. To invite the reemergence of traumatic histories of affective intensity and pitch without being swallowed up and destroyed" (p. 714). Almost from the beginning of increasing the treatment, Harper associated to me as the intrusive, overbearing mother, to whom closeness signaled actual abandonment and neglect. I had moved from being a fairly benign and helpful therapist to an object that posed a threat by its very closeness. I, on the other hand, accessed a deeper need in myself to be validated, and the ways in which we internalized our mothers and the ways they occupied our internal worlds as withholding presences led us to enact silences in the treatment. "What is unsymbolized," McGleughlin (2015) argued, "hides, erupts, displaces, confuses, creating interruptions, leaving gaps" (p. 214). She questioned whether "closing the gaps is the therapeutic ambition," rather than "inviting a kind of being with that might require the calling up and baring one's own gaps and ghosts" (p. 215).

Reflecting on the course of treatment required me to delve within myself to discover a part I both avoided and disowned. Significantly, our relationship changed. It did not begin with the resolution of a major enactment or sudden insight into what had been occurring between us in the analysis. "Therapeutic action," Harris (2009) pointed out, "and the breaking up of impasse, can occur through very minute shifts in the dyad or the individuals" (p. 6). The shifting self-state in me initiated something in Harper that allowed for an openness and receptivity to me as her therapist, to use me as a good object, in short, to become available to her, as we were no longer oscillating between a configuration of doer and done to (Benjamin, 2004).

As I moved from being a critical, demanding figure to a thoughtful, reflective one, and from a frustrated and irritated therapist to an empathic one, Harper, sensing my subtle shifting states, shifted as well from a fearful, withholding state to a more open and receptive one. Harper was gradually able to let go of her loyalty to old ties and release herself from an unending mourning process to accept her unspoken need for a good object relationship in the present. She began to use me as a benign and potentially benevolent presence. I was able to contain, metabolize, and transform the toxic introjects and projections from Harper's internal world, returning them to her in a more acceptable and benign manner. I could begin to speak from the absence I had created, and Harper was able to take in my detoxified projections through my ability to shift from my critical self-state to an empathic and maternal one. These changes, of course, were subliminal and unconscious, only emerging in the moment where she recognized and could speak from her need for the relationship. As McGleughlin (2015) suggested, "one needs to speak to the traumatized person from within the site of one's own trauma, rather than from an identification based on the recognition that each has experienced trauma" (p. 233).

Concurrent with reflecting on how the changes in our internal states evoked silence, absence, and reparation, I had an additional realization. Considering Davies's (2004) assertion that an impasse in the treatment is linked to an impasse in mourning in the analyst, led to my finally coming to understand this missing piece in our work.

Trauma speaks to trauma

After hearing a presentation by Adrienne Harris (2015), I began to think about the benign manner in which ghosts enter the consulting room through absence and silence. According to Kalb (2015), "ghosts are … reluctant ancestors" (p. 74). They are "internalizations gone awry" (Kalb, 2015, p. 74.) Thus, Harper was showing, not telling, her traumatic experience. When she came into treatment she was mourning the death of her father, and he, like most ghosts, did not "grow or change" (Kalb, 2015, p. 86), but haunted the border, the liminal space between past and present. Kalb speculated that ghosts were underrepresented aspects of early object relationships; " … inchoate, spectral, eerie, unburied, and undead psychic imprints that colonize body and soul" (p. 83). The late French psychoanalyst, Jean-Max Gaudilliere was fond of saying, "Trauma speaks to trauma" (quoted in Caruth, 2014, p. 307). What trauma did Harper and I share? Who were our ghosts that we shared? I located a shared experience with Harper—we each had a highly critical and demanding mother to whom we might seem less than visible—but it was not until I began to reflect on the progress of this treatment that I found another ghost who lurked in my history—a long absent and silent father. So, I realized, this also was a story about losses unmourned, and mourning that does not cease, and about the interaction between my history and hers. These figures needed to be laid to rest so that what was silenced could finally be spoken.

A forgotten piece of my history suddenly came to mind as I was revisiting my work with Harper. After my first marriage ended, I removed my wedding ring, but my ring finger felt uncomfortably bare. From a collection of rings that I have, I chose a simple ruby ring set in gold that had belonged to my father, and I wore it until I remarried. I never gave much thought to the significance of the ring. What about my father was I carrying with me, unconsciously and unintegrated? His own history was fraught with losses and disappointments. Because he was forced to work at age 13 to help support the family, any form of education was foreclosed to him. He often spoke of a wish to be a teacher and encouraged my interest in art and literature by providing books and art supplies. I did not go to college until I was 20, several years after my father died. Then, I was driven to succeed, to accumulate several advanced degrees, to teach, to write and publish papers, to undertake and complete analytic training, as if this were my destiny. Amazed by the revelation that some part of me was unconsciously living out my father's unlived life, his hopes and aspirations, I began to access the aspects of my relationship with my father that seemed unformulated or dissociated. I believe this realization impacted Harper's pathological mourning. McGleughlin (2015) asserted that if we were "willing … to struggle with our own internal splits to reach the other, a channel toward change and transformation may open … that impasse may loosen when the analyst … is able to metabolize, shift, grieve, change, and speak from this slightly altered state" (pp. 233–234).

The deeper trauma that Harper and I shared was the loss of our fathers. She openly and consciously mourned hers. I, on the other hand, lived out the trauma split off, unmourned, and unconscious of its effects. She longed to keep her father alive, whereas I wished to bring mine back to life. I am reminded of Davies's (1999) reflection on why we do analytic work, "to repair our ailing internal objects and heal ourselves and keep healing ourselves" (p. 187).

In a sense Harper and I have both been transformed by the therapeutic work. I do not remember the point at which I noticed that Harper rarely, if ever, wore her father's ring. It disappeared in those months when her life seemed to be falling apart, and we worked toward restructuring it.

One wintery night not long after our therapeutic work seemed to be on track again, I opened the door to greet Harper for her evening session. She entered dragging something dark and heavy behind her. It was long and black and looked like an iron dog. "What is that?" I exclaimed. "It looks like a dog." "It is," she replied. "I have been meaning to give it to you. It's an antique; it was my grandmother's." "What is it for?" I queried. "You put it outside," she said, "so people can wipe their feet. It's a mud scraper." I could barely contain my thoughts about the symbolism of the gift. It was dark and heavy, hard to carry, but it had stood the test of time and was moving from Harper's history into our shared experience.

Conclusions

The progress of this treatment illustrates and underscores the value and necessity of working long-term with trauma. Initially, I focused my investigation into Harper's relational difficulty by examining her relationship with her mother and attempting to provide a maternal response to her difficulties. Even though I realized that Harper's incomplete mourning process was central to her difficulties with interpersonal relationships and colored our interactions, I needed to locate an unmourned present absence in my own history to shift the internal work. While I was able to disclose the parallel in our experiences of the loss of our father, I had completely forgotten the existence of my father's ring and my own disavowal of the symbolism of the ring, partially as they predated my work as a therapist.

All treatments contain complexities that need to be identified, teased out, and integrated into the treatment. When I was able to finally mourn my melancholy object, Harper too could begin to let go of hers.

References

Aron, L. (1991). The patient's experience of the analyst's subjectivity. *Psychoanalytic Dialogues*, *1*(1), 29–51. doi:10.1080/10481889109538884.

Benjamin, J. (2004). Beyond doer and done to: An intersubjective view of thirdness. *Psychoanalytic Quarterly*, *73*(1), 5–46. doi:10.1002/j.2167-4086.2004.tb00151.x.

Caruth, C. (2014). *Listening to trauma: Conversations with leaders in the theory and treatment of catastrophic experience: Interviews and photography by Cathy Caruth*. Baltimore, MD: Johns Hopkins University Press.

Davies, J. M. (1999). Getting cold feet, defining "safe-enough" borders: Dissociation, multiplicity, and integration in the analyst's experience. *Psychoanalytic Quarterly*, *68*(2), 184–208. doi:10.1002/j.2167-4086.1999.tb00530.x.

Davies, J. M. (2004). Whose bad objects are we anyway? Repetition and our elusive love affair with evil. *Psychoanalytic Dialogues*, *14*(6), 711–732. doi:10.1080/10481881409348802.

Frosh, S. (2013). *Hauntings: Psychoanalysis and ghostly transmissions*. London: Palgrave Macmillan.

Grand, S. and Salberg, J. (2017). *Trans-generational trauma and the other: Dialogues across history and difference*. London: Routledge.

Harris, A. (2009). You must remember this. *Psychoanalytic Dialogues*, *19*(1), 2–21. doi:10.1080/10481880802634537.

Harris, A. (2015, February). *Ghosts in the 21st century consulting room*. Paper presented at a meeting of the Chicago Center for Psychoanalysis, Chicago, IL.

Harris, A., Kalb, M. and Klebanoff, S. (2016). *Ghosts in the consulting room: Echoes of trauma in psychoanalysis.* London: Routledge.

Kalb, M. (2015). Ghosts in the consulting room: Reluctant ancestors. *Contemporary Psychoanalysis*, *51*(1), 74–196. doi:10.1080/00107530.2015.985905.

McGleughlin, J. (2015). Do we find or lose ourselves in the negative? *Psychoanalytic Dialogues*, *25*(2), 214–236. doi:10.1080/10481885.2015.1013838.

Mitchell, S. A. (1988). *Relational concepts in psychoanalysis: An integration.* Cambridge, MA: Harvard University Press.

Salberg, J. and Grand, S. (2017). *Wounds of history: Repair and resilience in the trans-generational transmission of trauma.* London: Routledge.

Chapter 7

The role of ethnicity and culture in the long-term treatment of childhood trauma

Shoshana Ringel

Y started therapy approximately nine years ago, and we continue to meet currently, though on a less frequent basis. We initially met weekly to discuss current challenges in her life, but three years into the treatment, our focus shifted as we started to examine and process Y's traumatic history. Following this phase of intensive treatment, Y learned to observe repetitive patterns of relating to self and others, and to hold affective space from triggering events and interactions, gradually transforming her habitual ways of relating and becoming gentler with herself. In the final two years of treatment, we started to meet monthly, as Y would email me when she wished to process particular issues that had come up, and evoked her old destructive patterns. However, as Y herself stated, her problems became the challenges associated with privilege, rather than survival, such as difficulties with her doctoral studies, or conflicts with her upper class in-laws, concerns that she could never have imagined only a few years ago.

Although we ended up engaging in a long-term treatment, sometimes several times a week, Y. did not come to therapy seeking analysis, was not aware that the treatment was psychodynamic in nature, and certainly did not know that I was an analyst. However, many psychoanalytic elements were present, including the exploration of Y's familial history and its effect on her relationship to self and others, unconscious processes that shaped her behavior and motivation, and transference/countertransference dynamics that took place between the two of us. Unlike a more traditional psychoanalytic treatment structure that follows the prescribed frame of a 50-minute hour at consistent time intervals, our therapeutic process was far more fluid and flexible, eventually including Y's family members and consisting of longer sessions if necessary. Unlike the traditional psychoanalytic norms, we often hugged at the end of sessions.

While many psychoanalytic narratives of long-term treatment describe a traditional treatment frame and procedures, two accounts come to mind that did not follow the familiar analytic parameters and thus seem to me to correspond more closely to the treatment I describe in this chapter. Wiesel-Barth writes of her work with a long-term patient, which continued over several decades. During this time, she intervened following her patient's suicide attempts, arranged summer camp for the patient's daughter and, at times, paid her carfare. She also accompanied her patient to hospital and attended several important events in the patient's life (Wiesel-Barth, 2011). Clearly, the treatment went far beyond the traditional boundaries of patient/analyst relationship. Another account was written by the patient, rather than the analyst. In a June 2, 2015 *New York Times* blog series called "Couch", Gordon Marino, one of Beebe's patients described their analytic relationship, also decades long and mostly long-distance following his relocation across the country. He described how the therapy helped save his marriage, provided him support as a father and facilitated his studies and professional success. Marino offered a loving tribute to Beebe who became his friend and mentor in addition to being his trusted therapist, and to whom he could turn during challenging times in his life. Similarly, Y frequently told me how much she appreciated our work, and that I provided her with invaluable help, insights and support during challenging times in her life. For Y, I was a familiar other with whom she could identify, an immigrant like herself. Based on my own personal experience, I could understand her struggle to overcome poverty and hardship, to create a new life, and to belong. There was an element of mutual recognition between us that contributed to an immediate positive transference, as Benjamin describes in her writings, of both mutuality and difference (Benjamin, 2017). Though I was also an immigrant from another culture, I represented a new object, a possibility for a new relationship in the sense that I had achieved what Y's parents and family members could not, and would become her mentor, someone she could look up to, and a model for her own academic and professional aspirations. From the very beginning, I recognized that ours could not be a traditional treatment, and decided to be responsive to her emergent needs. Knowing that in the Chinese cultural system family was a significant factor in the individual's sense of identity and belonging, I agreed to meet with Y's husband to help negotiate relational difficulties, and with her brother and sister-in-law on several occasions to help resolve familial ruptures.

As I write this chapter, I wonder why certain patients remain in treatment for long periods of time. I reflect on the nature of change in the patient/therapist relationship over time and wonder if it may signify that cultural history and notions of self, family and social norms have played a significant role in determining the nature and evolution of this particular treatment.

Self, other and cultural context

Y decided to pursue treatment in her thirties following a series of conflicts with her supervisors at work, and chose me as her therapist when she discovered that I was an immigrant as well. From the beginning, I was drawn to Y's vivaciousness, spontaneity and earnestness. As she sprawled unselfconsciously among shawls and pillows on my couch, she seemed open and uninhibited in her behavior and emotional expression. She offered me her insights, sent me links to online articles, and suggested self-help books that she thought might help me to better understand her. It took a long time for Y to admit the extent of the physical and psychological abuse she had suffered at the hands of her father, aunt and grandmother.

During the first three years of treatment, our work was supportive in nature. We focused on Y's professional and interpersonal challenges, her mistreatment by supervisors, current conflicts with family members, and disappointments in social relationships. I validated her feelings and encouraged her to trust her own perceptions, to speak up and to protest the injustices done to her despite her fear that she was responsible, and that she would be severely punished if she dared to protest. At times, Y would look at me and ask if she really had permission to express her anger or to mourn her past. Was it OK for her to feel fear, grief and sadness, or was it merely an indulgence? Y had learned to view these emotions or any expression of "neediness" as weak and worthy of contempt. Whenever she expressed her outrage or sadness, Y would laugh and cover her face, minimizing the extent of her pain and embarrassed at her weakness. I encouraged Y to be gentler with herself and to learn to accept her fear, shame and vulnerability.

Y's sense of unworthiness and her powerful need to accommodate familial demands had deep roots in her Chinese culture and the Confucian worldview, a philosophical perspective that endorses social hierarchies, deference to patriarchal authority, and the predominance of familial systems over individual needs and personal identity (Tung, 1991; Wei-Ming, 1985). Y experienced intense conflict between her traditional Chinese upbringing, and the American values she was exposed to, which legitimized personal autonomy, subjective expression and self-actualization (Cushman, 1986). Western psychoanalytic paradigms have traditionally viewed the individual self as a central construct of human development (Kohut, 1977), and the development of cohesive self-organization has been a fundamental concern in self-psychology (Cushman, 1986). More recently, however, psychoanalytic perspectives have started to address the interface of sociocultural and political dimensions in self-other development, and to explore how these may impact the intrapsychic and the intersubjective domain of the analytic dyad (Brothers & Lewis, 2012; Dimen, 2011, as well as others).

Unlike the Western emphasis on subjectivity and differentiation, the Confucian concept of self is collectivist in nature, emphasizing social and familial harmony over self-expression and personal fulfillment. Individuals are expected to fulfill traditional gender roles within the social and familial system, and children are expected to obey their parents (Wei-Ming, 1985). Roland (1987, 1995) differentiates between the familial self, a self that is subject to hierarchical relationships, and the individualized self, which has been an exclusively Western construct until relatively recently. The Confucian system has offered a stable, although perhaps restrictive, social paradigm in China for millennia. However, the process of immigration and acculturation for many, including Y's family, has caused significant familial ruptures and interpersonal conflicts that have destabilized these traditional social structures.

Clinical history

Y came to the United States with her parents and younger brother at the age of seven. Her parents struggled for many years to survive and achieve financial stability, often uprooting Y from school in order to follow her father's unsuccessful financial schemes. From an early age, Y was required to become her parents' translator and facilitator in interactions with social service agencies, landlords and business owners. She also became her younger brother's caregiver, learning to put her own needs aside in order to take care of him and accommodate his demands. Y remembered that on one of her birthdays, her parents took her to buy a beautiful pair of boots that she had been longing for. However, her brother threw a tantrum and the family tried to appease him by buying him a gift first. By the time they returned to the shoe store, the boots were gone. Though Y was overcome by sadness and resentment as she was telling me the story, she minimized and dismissed her feelings. This was emblematic of her belief that she didn't matter, and shouldn't attach such significance to something so inconsequential that happened long ago.

Y's family, especially her father, utilized shame as a mechanism for the control and subjugation of younger and more vulnerable family members, especially women. Consequently, Y learned that it was safer to hide any signs of weakness or vulnerability, and to dissociate memories of the abuse and mistreatment she had experienced at the hand of her father and other relatives. She developed a fearful and ambivalent relationship with her volatile father. Y craved his love and validation, but was fearful of his unpredictable rage and violence. When he was in a good mood her father could be playful, but would suddenly become angry, lash out and hit her. When Y tried to ask him for something she wanted, or expressed an opinion, he would shame, humiliate and beat her. Y learned to keep her distance and to disavow her need for his love and affection. She believed that her father viewed her as a "beast of burden" whose only value lay in working for him and bailing him out whenever his ill-conceived ventures failed. Shaw describes what he calls "traumatic narcissism", which stems from intergenerational trauma, as a "delusional infallibility and entitlement", the "externalizing of shame", and the "suppression of the subjectivity of the other" (Shaw, 2014, p. 35). In response to her father's violence and narcissism, Y abandoned her own authentic self, taking on his burden of shame and humiliation (Davies, 2004; Fairbairn, 1952). By internalizing and identifying with the narcissistic parent's shaming and abuse, the child sustains the hope for love and validation from the traumatizing parent (Davies & Frawley, 1993).

Y's father carried his own trauma in the aftermath of poverty, violence and famine in China during his childhood and adolescence, the loss of family members and siblings to disease, and his own mother's emotional and physical abuse of him. The pattern of longing for paternal love and acceptance was repeated in Y's romantic pursuit of unavailable men who rejected and mistreated her. Y shared with me a Chinese proverb that encapsulates her futile quest for love: "You keep banging on the locked treasure chest hoping to find gold, but you find only a nugget". Not surprisingly, we recognized that her father's volatile temper and disdain of weakness or vulnerability in others were often activated within Y in response to others whom she viewed as weak and vulnerable.

Unlike her father, Y's mother was kind and loving, though she was also childlike and intellectually limited. Her mother's love and support for her sustained Y throughout her childhood, but she could not turn to her for mentoring or protection. Y remembered a folktale her mother used to tell her that went as follows:

> There was a poor mother and son in Imperial China. At the time, the only way for the poor to succeed in China was to pass the imperial civil examinations. After rigorous studies, the son succeeded in passing the exams and he became a magistrate. He returned home dressed in his shining new robes, but his mother could not recognize him. He called "Mother! Mother!" and she finally realized that her son had returned in glory, and that her dream came true.

As Y was telling me the story, she started to cry. I asked why she was sad, and Y replied: "Not sad, happy, my mother's dream for me will also come true, and I will return home, dressed in my doctoral cap and gown just as she had envisioned". Indeed, Y eventually achieved her dream, traditionally reserved for Chinese sons, and though she was a girl, and treated as an inferior member in her family, she ultimately far surpassed her brother both academically and professionally. After his death she became her parents' only surviving, and therefore treasured, child. In her relationship with her mother, Y took on alternating roles of child and parent, dependent and caregiver, struggling to maintain boundaries and to claim her own identity.

Y's conflicting desires to be loved through submission and accommodation versus her quest to attain independence and autonomy were enacted in our relationship. At times, Y wanted to be a child, asking me for hugs, advice, and permission to express her emotions. At other times, she asserted her independence, setting her own terms for the time and date of our sessions. In the transference/countertransference, I was the nurturing, loving mother who was also someone Y could look up to and idealize. I could tolerate separation and uncertainty while, unlike her mother, I didn't need Y to take care of me. With me, Y could find her own voice and learn to set boundaries, and I became her safe haven to return to as she was creating a new life for herself.

As she grew older, Y started to resent her parents' and brother's increased reliance on her, but it was difficult for her to assert her own limits. We both recognized she was up against thousands of years of culture and tradition. Y had been raised to obey and serve while staying quiet and invisible, "kept in the closet". It took her years to reveal to me the extent of the physical and emotional abuse she had suffered at the hands of her father and relatives, and to own and express her pain and anger. Having learned that tenderness and vulnerability were to be despised, shame kept her from admitting her abuse to others and from showing me her pain.

Disorganized attachment

Disorganized attachment is activated when the stability of the child/caregiver system is undermined by anxiety, fear and shame (Slade, 2014; Sroufe, 2009). Children, who depend on their caregiver for safety and survival, are highly vigilant to any survival threat, especially a threat to their primary attachment system upon which their safety and security are founded (Slade, 2014). Fear, a predominant emotion in disorganized attachment, is triggered as a response to parental threat or abandonment, but also when the parent's unresolved trauma is transmitted to the child, often implicitly, in the form of fearful anxiety (Beebe, Lachmann, Markese & Bahrick, 2012; Bowlby, 1963; Lyons-Ruth, Dutra, Schuder & Bianchi, 2006).

In Y's family, traumatic narratives were passed from one generation to the next through physical and verbal abuse, and through poverty, disease and death. Some of the indices of disorganized adult attachment include denial and minimization of the abuse, self-blame, confusion of the self with the perpetrator, and a highly detailed memory of the traumatic event. Adult attachment interviews of disorganized/disoriented speakers suggest imagistic, sensory and affective memories which are fragmented and frozen in time (Hesse, 2008; Hesse & Main, 2000). Following traumatic events, particularly childhood trauma associated with abuse and neglect, one may develop strategies for containing and compartmentalizing unbearable memories and affects through fragmented self-states. These self-states are structured to keep the full extent of the trauma, which is deeply embedded in early, often nonverbal and implicit experience, hidden and dissociated from the patient's conscious memory (Bromberg, 2006).

The traumatic transmission from parent to child may occur when the parent, rather than soothing and comforting the child during times of distress, withdraws or becomes punitive. The child then learns that expressing their needs is dangerous and may result in the parent's withdrawal, rejection or active retaliation. Children therefore learn to hide their vulnerability through aggressive behaviors or through compliance and accommodation (Brandschaft, Doctors & Sorter, 2010). According to attachment research, disorganized children, whose attachment patterns are based on fear and shame, do not develop a sense of felt security based on ongoing and meaningful affective experiences with their caregivers and do not learn to regulate their affective states (Lyons-Ruth et al., 2006). Y was taught to ignore and reject her subjective experience and to accommodate her father and older relatives who carried their own disavowed and unresolved loss and trauma.

Shame is closely associated with a disorganized attachment system (Sroufe, 2009), and is a powerful affect that is typically related to interpersonal trauma. Shaming has been found to be a potent weapon used by the adult perpetrator to control and dominate, and is a particularly effective method for subjugating women (Lewis, 1971, 1987). It was utilized by Y's father and older relatives to control and silence her, and her shame became a habitual response to perceived failure, rejection and disappointment.

Working through Y's childhood trauma

The treatment shifted when Y's brother became seriously ill. This painful experience triggered traumatic memories from Y's childhood that she had previously dissociated or ignored. During the following year, we worked through her grief, anger and guilt related to her brother's illness and eventual death. Dissociated self-states that Y had denied and silenced emerged and fragments of her traumatic history gradually became more accessible. Y described holding her brother in her arms as he lay dying, as if he was her child. He was terrified of dying, holding on to Y as he was struggling to breathe. Though they were able to make peace before he died, images of his final hours continued to haunt Y in nightmares and flashbacks, and his death seemed to release affects and memories that had long been dormant. Y could no longer hold her memories of abuse and trauma at bay and they flooded in. She started to express anger at her father's and relatives' mistreatment of her throughout her childhood, and later at her brother's selfishness and repeated betrayals (he never stood up for her, and would side with her abusive relatives against her).

As we processed her grief, anger and sadness, Y and I discovered that her frequent conflicts with supervisors and co-workers had deep roots in her relationships with her father and extended family. She felt trapped in a cycle of fear and resentment towards those in authority who had mistreated her, but was helpless to protest because she felt shame at her perceived failure and incompetence. Y's conflicts with others revealed a pattern of subjugation and accommodation in response to criticism and rejection. We realized how addictive this pattern was, and that hurt and betrayal had become her relational home, the emotional place she retreated to, and what she expected and even sought. The pain felt familiar and comforting.

During one of our sessions, Y mourned her lost childhood and her isolation. She was the outsider, both in her extended family and among her school peers. We explored how her fear was activated with her violent and shaming father, and how Y responded to his violence by "freezing", "enduring" and "playing dead" like a frightened animal, unable to risk infuriating him and eliciting retaliation.

As our work continued, other dissociated affects and self-states that Y had silenced started to emerge. One of the more significant was the frightened, isolated little girl who didn't trust anyone and who preferred to hide in the pain and darkness that she was familiar with. I recognized the little girl part when Y's voice softened and became childlike. She would then hide under a shawl or cover her face in her hands, too embarrassed to have me witness her fear and vulnerability. During one of our sessions, I saw this child part emerging in Y's voice and facial expression, and asked her to tell me who she was. Y answered "We don't want you to know". Y was shocked and embarrassed, she was not aware of how alive this child self was within her. As we processed this interaction Y became aware that she was protecting her child self from my intrusion and from potential harm. Her child part did not trust me; she was frightened of coming out and being seen by me. Y explained to me that her little girl self preferred to remain hidden in darkness, surrounded by the familiar pain, where she was lonely but safe and secure. Y's desire to protect herself from my potential impingements may have been enacted between us as she eventually started to maintain a safe distance from me by maintaining control of the frequency and times for sessions, as if letting me know that the treatment would only take place on her own terms.

As our work continued, states of shame and guilt emerged as well. Harsh internal voices flooded Y whenever she tried to protest or disclose mistreatment by family and others. She would tell me that after sessions she could spend hours in bed, overwhelmed by traumatic memories and affects and unable to function. But she was determined to confront her inner demons before becoming herself a mother, so as not to transmit the pattern of abuse and shame to her own child. We recognized that Y had difficulty disentangling from internalized rage and harsh self-judgements, that her states of shame and self-hatred had a powerful pull on her. Pain was familiar and comforting and Y was afraid to believe that love and freedom were reliable or lasting. After every step towards freeing herself and loosening the bonds, the voices became louder and more insistent. Y was trained to dismiss and reject her fear and sadness, and responded harshly towards any sign of her own helplessness and vulnerability.

As Y's relationship to more vulnerable parts of herself continued to unfold, she started to report a gradual change in her relationship to others for whom she could now experience more empathy and compassion. She was becoming more aware of danger signals, so that she was able to distance herself from toxic relationships and destructive interactions. With time, Y was learning to hold and accept states of fear and helplessness, and rather than reflexively withdraw into her familiar pain or punish herself with self-judgements, she was learning to be more gentle and kind with herself, and to regulate a range of affects through empathic explorations between the two of us. As I accompany her on her journey, I hold and envision a different future for her that includes love and respect, but I have also learned not to impinge or intrude, and to allow Y time and space to find her own voice (Grossmark, 2012).

Reflections on our long-term treatment

During the intensive processing of Y's traumatic history we met several times a week. After about a year, there was a gradual tapering off of frequency of sessions. Y was coming into her own as an adult and as a professional as she pursued her doctoral studies and obtained her PhD, and as she started to consider becoming a mother. During the past two years, a new pattern was established between us where Y would call me when she was experiencing a crisis, or when old destructive patterns were triggered following interactions with family members or friends, and she needed further processing and integration. But mostly, Y wanted to become her own person and to handle her difficulties on her own, and she would come to therapy only as a last resort. Y did let me know how much she appreciated my help and the work we had done together, and I understood her desire to strike out on her own and to develop her autonomy and self-reliance while knowing that I would be there if she needed me. Unlike with her mother, we could be close without a need for merger, and she would use our relationship to practice differentiation and assertiveness without the fear of retaliation (as with her father) or recriminations (as with her mother).

As I reflect on our relationship, I feel a deep regard and affection for Y. She has grown a great deal and we have become quite close over the years. Both of us grew up in working class immigrant families, were excluded by peers, and relied on academic achievements to find our niche and to fit in, and therefore many aspects of her history felt quite familiar. As her therapist, I deeply appreciated Y's motivation and determination to face her painful childhood trauma and to process our work on her own between sessions, working hard to gain understanding and to bring about change and transformation in her life. When I met her family and witnessed her brother's illness and eventual death, I felt as if I had become an honorary member of her family (he came to sessions with an oxygen tank, barely able to breathe or talk). At times, however, I found our relationship quite frustrating. Although we discussed Y's need for autonomy and self-reliance, in part through having considerable control over the frequency and timing of our sessions, I still found it difficult at times to tolerate not knowing when I would hear from her, or find the flexibility to accommodate her whenever she contacted me requesting a session. I had to learn to relinquish control, and accept uncertainty and trust that the work will take place in its own way. The unpredictability of our sessions during the past couple of years evoked my own difficulty with separations and reunions and ultimately taught me to accept Y's developmental needs despite my own insecurities. As stated previously, I reflect that while to some extent our relationships mirrors Y's relationship with her mother, it has also become a new relational pattern that allows her to experience a close bond and still maintain a measure of autonomy and independence.

Conclusion

In this chapter, I described how, because of powerful cultural traditions and the challenges of growing up in a poor immigrant family, Y learned to submit and accommodate to others and to hide her own fear and vulnerability as she negotiated her personal and professional path. Gradually, Y overcame the burden of fear and shame, and learned to recognize and accept vulnerable internal states that she, and others, had silenced and disavowed. She developed a deeper empathy for those traumatized parts of herself so that these could be heard and integrated.

As I reflect on the years that we have spent together, I recognize that beyond our patient/therapist relationship, Y looked to me to provide what her parents were unable or unprepared to give. They had lived in a different era, a tumultuous cultural period in China when parents could not protect their children from hardships, and where higher education and life choices were not available for the poor. Y's mother was illiterate and could not teach her how to engage and succeed in a Western world, develop relationships and get along with supervisors and co-workers. Her parents could not understand and provide support for her professional aspirations. In addition to my role as a therapist who helped Y work through her difficult history, I also became a role model and a mentor. My roots in a different culture, and my own experience as an immigrant, helped me recognize Y's struggle to construct her identity, speak a different language, and navigate a bicultural self.

During a recent session, Y again discussed old patterns of negative self-judgements that had been triggered following the completion of her doctoral program and then as she became pregnant. She wasn't fully able to take in her successes and achievements, which she had worked so hard to attain. Instead, she returned again and again to the familiar place of fear and shame, believing that she didn't deserve her success, that if she allowed herself to feel joy everything would fall apart. However, this time around Y was able to observe the familiar sequence with more equanimity, and to eventually disengage from these familiar mental loops.

References

Beebe, B., Lachmann, F., Markese, S. and Bahrick, L. (2012). On the origins of disorganized attachment and internal working models: Paper I: A dyadic systems approach. *Psychoanalytic Dialogues, 22*(2), 253–272.

Benjamin, J. (2017). *Beyond doer and done to: Recognition theory, intersubjectivity and the third.* New York, NY: Routledge.

Bowlby, J. (1963). Pathological mourning and childhood mourning. *Journal of the American Psychoanalytic Association, 11*, 500–541.

Brandschaft, B., Doctors, S. and Sorter D. (2010). *Toward an emancipatory psychoanalysis: Brandschaft's intersubjective vision.* New York, NY: Routledge.

Bromberg, P. (2006). *Awakening the dreamer: Clinical journeys.* Hillsdale, NJ: Analytic Press.

Brothers, D. and Lewis, J. (2012). Homesickness, exile, and the self-psychological language. *International Journal of Psychoanalytic Self Psychology, 7*(2), 180–195. Bantam.

Cushman, P. (1986). *Constructing the self, constructing America.* New York, NY: Addison Wesley.

Davies, J.M. (2004). Whose bad objects are we anyway? Repetition and our elusive love affair with evil. *Pscyhonalytic Dialogues, 14*, 711–732.

Davies, J. and Frawley, M.G. (1993). *Treating the adult survivor of childhood sexual abuse: A psychoanalytic perspective.* New York, NY: Basic Books.

Dimen, M. (2011). *With culture in mind.* New York, NY: Routledge.

Fairbairn, D. (1952). *Psychoanalytic studies of the personality.* London: Tavistock Pubs.

Grossmark, R. (2012). The unobtrusive relational analyst. *Psychoanalytic Dialogues, 22*, 629–646.

Hesse, E. (2008). The adult attachment interview: Protocol, methods of analysis, and empirical studies. In J. Cassidy & P. Shaver (Eds.), *Handbook of attachment*, pp. 552–598. New York, NY: Guilford.

Hesse, E. and Main, M. (2000). Disorganized infant, child, and adult attachment: Collapse in behavioral and attentional strategies. *Journal of the American Psychoanalytic Association, 48*(4), 1097–1127.

Kohut, H. (1977). *The restoration of the self.* New York, NY: International Universities Press.

Lewis, H.B. (1971). *Shame and guilt in neurosis.* New York, NY: International Universities Press.

Lewis, H.B. (1987). *The role of shame in symptom formation.* Hillsdale, NJ: Erlbaum.

Lyons-Ruth, K., Dutra, L., Schuder, M. and Bianchi, I. (2006). From infant attachment disorganization to adult dissociation: Relational adaptations or traumatic experiences? *Psychiatric Clinics of North America, 29*, 63–86.

Roland, A. (1987). The familial self, the individualized self, and the transcendent self: Psychoanalytic reflections on India and America. *Psychoanalytic Review, 74*(2), 237–250.

Roland, A. (1995). How universal is the psychoanalytic self? In M. Perez-Foster, M. Moskowitz & R. Javier (Eds.), *Reaching across boundaries of culture and class*, pp. 71–90. New York, NY: Jason-Aronson Inc.

Shaw, D. (2014). *Traumatic narcissism: Relational system of subjugation*. New York, NY: Routledge.

Slade, H. (2014). Imagining fear: Attachment, threat and psychic experience. *Psychoanalytic Dialogues*, *24*(3), 253–266.

Sroufe, L.A. (2009). The concept of development in developmental psychopathology. *Child Development Perspectives*, *3*, 178–183.

Tung, M. (1991). Insight oriented psychotherapy and the Chinese patient. *American Journal of Orthopsychiatry*, *61*(2), 186–194.

Wei-Ming, T. (1985). Selfhood and otherness in Confucian thought. In A. Marsella, G. DeVos & F. Hsu (Eds.), *Culture and self*, pp. 331–351. New York, NY: Tavistock Pubs.

Wiesel-Barth, J. (2011). Katherine: A long hard case. *International Journal of Self Psychology*, *6*(4), 444–468.

Chapter 8

It takes a long time to grow young

Working relationally with developmental trauma

Natalie Peacock-Corral

As I enter Julia's home, a smell of cigarettes and wild animals knocks me over. Something went horribly wrong here. A child went missing, tragically in this very home; she was just a few years younger than I am when I enter. I look into the fireplace, spellbound by the wounded fox sitting there. I hear the sounds of an owl living in the back room. My mother's cousin, Julia, whose own mother is my namesake, puffs on her cigarettes and laughs heartily with damaged vocal chords. As a child, I don't question why anyone would live this way. I am not afraid to be in her home. I am fascinated. Like Julia I am drawn to healing the wounded. They don't scare me.

As I began to write this book chapter, this long-ago repressed memory from age ten resurfaced. Psychotherapists bring their own capacities and histories into the treatment. My life implicitly prepared me for being able to meet Robert and stay in treatment with him for 18 years.

We begin

In January of 2000, I meet Robert, aged 38, who is a Caucasian male, married with four children. As we begin, I am undaunted by his numerous psychiatric treatment failures, years of cannabis dependence, history of trauma, outbursts of uncontrollable rage, and utter lack of psychological mindedness. I have no idea of the task I am about to undertake.

Two years into our work, Robert talks about how he hates his job and feels guilty for taking so much sick leave. He feels trapped, anxious, victimized, and persecuted. He tells me, "I am happy being miserable. Life is like a prison sentence without parole. I am dead inside. When I smoke marijuana, it is the only time I feel relief." He describes himself as an "unmovable brick building." I imagine pushing on the building, but it doesn't move. No matter how I try to connect with him, he barrels forward with his ruminative despair. I feel helpless and utterly invisible. He holds me captive and he knows it. I viscerally feel I'm being strangled and find myself giving up. Pretending to be calm, I feel sedated, frozen. The clock moves much too slowly. To keep myself alive, I mentally exit the session, imagining myself a few hours later in my rehearsal for an opera, enraptured by the music of *The Merry Widow*.

Where did my compassion go? The therapist I am tonight is not the therapist who has been deeply moved by the desolation Robert describes himself feeling as he sits alone in his garage night after night. In winter, he shivers in the cold, inhales cannabis smoke, and coughs. Sometimes he smokes so heavily he vomits. He pinches his face to keep himself awake well past the time he should be sleeping for work the next day. If he delays sleep, he delays the next day of insurmountable work. If he stays awake, he doesn't have to face the false life he has, the job he despises, and his lack of qualifications. But his job is not the only thing he's trying to escape.

When Robert was ten, his mother broke her back, and then later developed muscular dystrophy. His father, who had polio as a child, needed crutches to walk. His father, abandoned by his own father, raised by a single mother who was part of a religious cult, lived in an iron lung for a year as a child. Although Robert had an accomplished sister two years his senior from whom he became estranged, he became his mother's primary caretaker until he left home as an adult. "I have to martyr myself for my family," he often says. "When will it be MY turn?"

Reverie of Robert as a child

I captured the feelings I have for the young Robert in a reverie that is based on his history although the setting is my own fabrication:

> Robert is running farther and farther into the woods, pushing himself, trying to run ahead of his mother's screams of pain. He can't catch his breath or stop thinking "I broke my mother's back. I made her sick." He runs in circles just as he did when he was four and his mother would tell him to stop. She can't stop him now; she is lying in a hospital bed in their home. He feels suddenly dizzy and begins to vomit violently. Falling into a soft patch of leaves under a towering tree, Robert is a small skinny 11-year-old with red hair, freckles, pale skin, and blue eyes. He knows he won't be missed even if he is gone for hours. His father will be relieved that he is not home causing trouble.
>
> Robert cannot erase the look of horror on his mother's face when she broke her back. He was just a few inches away, in the back seat of the car, behaving badly. His mother turned around to stop him and her spine snapped. She recovered and developed muscular dystrophy a year later. His father yells at him all the time now, telling him everyone's job is to take care of mother, who keeps getting worse. Where are the delicious meals, his favorite oatmeal cookies she once cooked for him, the school projects she made with him? At night, he crawls into his mother's hospital bed to sleep with her even though his skinny limbs press hard against the

cold bars of the bed. Her body is pained and rigid. He longs to feel her close and have her wrap herself around him as she did just two years ago.

Rage, not tears

When baby elephants lose their mothers, they will weep for hours. Some even die.

Robert never cried when his mother broke her back and got sick. Instead, he raged. He threw himself down a flight of stairs when he was ten. At 11 he cut himself superficially with a razor, lifting his shirt to show his parents. At 15, he beat another student unconscious and was sued by the victim's parents.

Even though his words spoke otherwise, Robert's father acted as if Robert were to blame for breaking his mother's back. His father made him climb dangerously high onto the roof to fix things and made him cut shrubbery for hours until his hands bled. Strong and agile, Robert could handle almost any punishing task his father gave him. He thought he deserved what he got because he was bad. Robert's father demanded he get all As in school. Afraid of failing, he would lie frozen in bed for hours as an adolescent, feigning physical illness.

He had repeated night terrors in which he was in a bowl of noodles, growing smaller as the noodles got bigger. In the dark of the night, he would be found shivering and terrified in a corner of his bedroom. He entered an excellent college early, majoring in physics as had his father, a professor of physics. By the time he was in his early twenties, he had transferred to six different colleges, eventually ending up with an associate's degree from a community college. The first of four babies was on the way with his 20-year-old wife, herself a victim of severe early abuse. Addicted to sex, Robert demanded intercourse up to ten times a day. Through sheer determination and raw talent, he built a successful career based on a false self that is in shambles when I meet him. Not surprisingly, two of his children have developed significant mental health issues.

From the beginning of our work together, I felt I was working with two different patients. When in crisis, Robert was a terror, his thinking was concrete, his regression palpable. He couldn't manage the basics of self-care and would often fly into a rage at the slightest provocation. Frequently in crisis, this is the Robert I first got to know. And yet I sensed another Robert in the room – intelligent, creative, even compassionate. He loved music as I did. Although rare, moments of softness emerged between us, remnants of the early connection he had with his mother. He loved to fix things at home and was a master woodturner although he rarely spoke about his craft. Skilled in the use of his favorite hammer, he often turned it against himself, beating his feet raw. Through 18 years of our work, Robert continued to show me both the builder and destroyer sides of his personality.

A different lens

Robert, to say the least, is a challenging patient for a young social worker. In the third year of our work, I enter an advanced psychoanalytic psychotherapy program and delve deeply into the writings of Freud, Kohut, Winnicott, Schaefer, Gabbard, Bettelheim, Mitchell, and Searles, among others. I will never forget the resonant feeling I have the evening we discuss sadomasochistic object relations and when I hear a fragment of a quote by Schaefer (2003), "… the patient's fears of their own benevolent feelings that would lead to giving up the paranoid and masochistic position from which they have been deriving security and perverse pleasure, even at the cost of conscious psychic pain." (p. 89). Now I have a framework to understand Robert's shifting sense of self. When I learn about using countertransference, projection, and projective identification in working with sadomasochism, I begin to understand my tortured experience with Robert through a different lens. My sense of deadness, of being trapped and strangled when I am with him, is a way to understanding, countertransferentially, what he feels inside (Schaefer, 2003; Searles, 1979).

I meet with a clinical supervisor, Judy, who is ferociously smart, tenacious, and tough. She respects my work, believes in me and my treatment with Robert. While I feel deadened and trapped in my sessions with Robert, I feel held and enlivened when I meet with Judy. Judy holds me as a therapist, which allows me to better hold Robert (Fraiberg, Adelson, & Shapiro, 1975; Winnicott, 1960).

Nailing floorboards

During a session five years in, Robert's declarations are all too familiar:

> I see myself dead. What is the point of living? I'm like a bum on the street. I see myself locked away in an institution for life. I'd rather move into a storage locker, where people put their belongings, where there are no windows.

I have a powerful association as he speaks, and share it with him. "I see you working with your hands in a home with vivid blue walls. The light is streaming in, and I see you nailing floorboards." I think of his building a floor for himself, and how I hold that vision for him before he can (Loewald, 1960).

My early interventions around self-care were not welcomed. Robert binged on big bags of candy and refused to eat healthy dinners his wife made for his family, although he was prediabetic and 40 pounds overweight. In the spirit of Kohut's empathic attunement (Kohut, 1971), I learned to time interventions around basic needs with the utmost attunement and a collaborative stance. After multiple adjunctive treatments (i.e., a substance-abuse group, a dialectical behavioral therapy (DBT) group, a top-notch 28-day dual disorders inpatient program, an anger management group, a meditation program, and other group psychotherapy work with a psychiatrist, and two short inpatient admissions), Robert dismisses their value and hands me the materials he obtained, saying, "You keep them. I don't need or want them. My real treatment is with you."

The kicking babies

Seven years into this challenging work, I became pregnant with my first child. Here is my description of a session during that time: Kick, kick, kick goes the baby inside me. I sit with Robert, my belly round and protruding, five months into my pregnancy. He lies down on the sofa, curls up towards the wall, swaddles himself in a blanket, and refuses to speak once again. Just 15 minutes ago after a long, hard swim, I was feeling joyous about the new life growing inside me. My baby settles and stops kicking. I sit with the silence in the room. Robert's back is turned to me. Finally, he says.

> I don't like our work lately. You are not helping me. I don't want to work in therapy. You are asking me to do work in here. I don't want to work in therapy. That's your job. I should be able to act anyway I want to in here. You can't ask me to do anything.

Kick, kick, kick goes the patient.

I look at him and imagine a baby screaming in his crib. I ask him to sit up and not turn away. "I need to see your eyes." Surprisingly, he sits up, his belly protruding under his ill-fitting shirt, tattoos covering his legs, his face locked in rage. "I wonder if you're having trouble with my pregnancy. As my belly grows, so does your anger, your absences from work, watching beheadings on the internet, sleeping all day, and locking yourself in your bedroom." "I haven't given the pregnancy a second thought," he counters. We sit in a prolonged silence, frozen. Instead of saying, "I want to be your baby. I want to be the baby inside of you," I hear him say the words he has spoken many times before, "That baby is such a lucky baby," as he drops his head down in sorrow.

After eight weeks of his relentless silence, unacknowledged longing, and rage, I feel I must wall myself off from him. I am unmoved by this moment of softness. What I want to do is kick, kick, kick the patient right now, kick him out of my office, be done with him, send him away for good. "Get away from me and my baby, you son of a bitch," I think to myself. The intensity of my thoughts startles me, but I don't care. "To hell with him." My clinical supervisor told me yesterday to "stick with it." If only she were in the room right now, she would know there is no way I can possibly endure this. In this moment, I decide this is where we will end.

That night I dream *I am on a bike on the side of a road and Robert is driving a car behind me with his wife in the passenger seat. His car bumps into me while his wife laughs at my unsteadiness, my attempts to keep cycling and not fall. I never let go of my bike, never fall, but I feel the fright in my body.* I know my bike is no match for my patient's car.

During my first pregnancy, *I also dream I am nursing Robert, and he bites my breast with sharp jagged teeth.* This was how I felt during the early stages of the treatment. I made multiple attempts to "feed" him, but instead of taking in my good milk, he bit me. Taking another bite, Robert decides he will leave treatment, letting me know by voicemail in a saddened tone. I tell Judy how difficulty this treatment is, and also consult with Heather, a highly respected psychoanalyst. Judy says, "Stick with it, Natalie!" Heather advises me to recognize my limits, especially now that I'm expecting my first child. Feeling I have a choice frees me, and I reluctantly contact Robert and ask him to come in to discuss his decision to leave. I feel conflicted about asking him to come in, conflicted about his continuing. He had kicked himself out before I could reject him. However, when we meet he chooses to return. Judy sticks with me, and I stick with Robert.

Robert and I are now seven years into our work, and a dream a patient shared with his analyst, Philip Bromberg, captures my feelings about Robert: "I [the patient] was leaning out of a window on the top floor of a tall building that was in flames. A fireman was climbing up a ladder to rescue me, and I was throwing rocks at him" (1998, p. 207). This patient's words could just as well be Robert's. He says, "I fully expect you to 'cure' me and I'm prepared to defeat you. I don't have an illness, I am my illness and I won't let you cure me of being who I am" (p. 208).

When I was on maternity leave, I suffered from four months of severe postpartum depression triggered by my difficulties with attempting to breastfeed my daughter. I learned what it means to be a psychiatric patient who is terrified. My experience of depression opened me up to experiencing a deeper empathic understanding of Robert.

Feeding therapy

Robert is clearly relieved when I return from maternity leave; he had seen a trusted colleague while I was away. Although a strong negative transference has marked the first seven years of our work, during the next two years an idealizing transference emerges. Earlier Robert often put me in the role of his father, stating, "I will be spanked in here no matter what I say." I was experienced as a dictatorial presence who threatened to end his cannabis use even though my approach was the opposite of this. Upon my return Robert describes therapy as "a form of eating, like food" and tells a colleague our treatment "is REAL therapy." He leaves me a note on a scrap of paper: "You're great" and stops fighting me at every turn. He can also acknowledge his attachment: "You are like family to me. This therapy is my WIFE. I heavily depend on this therapy." And he finally agrees to increase our number of sessions to several per week. Between my two pregnancies that were two years apart, I open another relational door by inviting Robert to leave voicemail messages between our sessions. I explain that I won't return his calls unless he indicates an urgent need. The process provides a containing function as he imagines me receiving his messages, and supports object constancy, as he hears my voice. Demonstrating a growing capacity to be more self-reflective, he uses voicemail as a reparative tool, container, and transitional object, by explaining, apologizing, taking ownership of, and reflecting upon his difficult behavior in a recent session. Sometimes he expresses his gratitude, which he rarely does in our sessions.

D.W. Winnicott joins us

Robert's hostile response to my second pregnancy mirrored his response to my first. However, during this time I am not alone in our treatment. D.W. Winnicott has joined us, (*and it isn't just for a cup of tea*). I hold in my mind the Winnicottian (1969) idea of surviving the patient's rage without retaliating. I carry a vision of myself: *I am a great mountain, able to endure many storms.* His spewing rage and hostile projections no longer rattle me. I am fiercely determined that his rage won't destroy me, my in utero baby, him, or our treatment.

This dream, which occurs during a brief enactment that is similar to one during my first pregnancy, reflects my state of mind during that time: *I dream I am on one side of a pyramid, attempting to get to the other side. Robert is shooting bullets at me with a BB gun. I know he won't kill me, but the bullets sting. I say to myself, "All I have to do is get to the other side of this."* My dream foreshadows how we get to the other side of my second pregnancy with some stinging moments that I know I can endure.

Working relationally: a breakthrough occurs

By the time of this pregnancy, I have taken courses that are far more relevant to Robert's treatment and read the work of Phillip Bromberg and Harold Searles. I continue with my relational psychoanalytically oriented peer supervision and individual supervision with Heather, a relationally oriented social worker/psychoanalyst. When I read Bromberg, a breakthrough occurs. Instead of seeing Robert exclusively through the lens of borderline personality disorder, I draw on an understanding of self-states, and disassociation as a response to trauma. I feel our sessions shift as I adopt a more relational stance (Bromberg, 1998; Mitchell & Black, 1995; Wallin, 2007). I draw attention to what is happening between us, for example, by saying, "You are really wanting to fight me right now. You feel bad inside and all you know how to do is pick a fight or stay silent. Let's try a different approach." Or "I feel helpless over here. When you speak in this way I feel very distanced from you." At times, he barrels forward without responding. At another point he says, "I feel distanced from myself when I am like that." It often takes multiple attempts before he softens and acknowledges what I say. When I verbalize during my second pregnancy how frightening my first pregnancy must have been, I speak directly to his fears: "I am not leaving you. I will be back after my maternity leave time, just like I was before." Robert knows I will stick by him. On my return from my second pregnancy, I sense the potential for both rupture and repair in our relationship reflected in a dream in which I am married to him. *There's a warmth between us. But spiders on the wall keep jumping off to bite me in the dream, causing painful welts.* Our closeness is not without peril.

Music as our secret garden

In our twelfth year together, Robert takes a relational leap in our treatment. In his family, he had kept his love of music under wraps. "I was closeted about it. I wanted it only for myself. I thought I was a bad child listening to bad music." He remembers his father using his crutches to knock down an elaborate play structure Robert had created, yelling "get to work and stop playing!" Robert felt guilty when he played, making it difficult for us to engage in play together. But when he makes a passing comment about his love of music, I leap upon the possibility to create a new collaborative relational experience (Stern, 2015). After some thought, I disclose to him how much I enjoy music and that I am a singer, which encourages him to reveal how much he loves music and how much he knows. He has an encyclopedic knowledge of classic rock and garage band punk music. I invite him to bring music into our sessions. Initially, he's cautious about the music he brings in, choosing pieces he imagines I will like. I delight in his offerings and talk excitedly about my experience of what he's brought. With more daring, he brings songs that mirror his inner experience, demonstrating that music is the royal road to his unconscious. He brings in such titles as "Orphan Boy," "Feeling Sad and Lonely," "Feeling Yourself Disintegrate," "This Ain't No Picnic," "Slit My Wrists," "Unsatisfied," "Hard to be Human Again," "Calm me Down," "My Confusion," "I Think I am Down," and "Night of the Sadist." "I could tell you my life story through words," he says, "or through music. Music would be the real story." But he doesn't comment directly on the stories of his music choices, nor do I, respecting the need to play without interpreting (Kohut, 1971; Winnicott, 1971). Joy, aliveness, an occasional sliver of humor, and, most profoundly, hope, now enter our play space once characterized by deadness and my feeling trapped in old patterns of sadomasochistic relating.

We listen to music in our sessions and Robert explains how his life parallels the troubled lives of many of the artists. With music he allows himself another form of grieving and speaks about his losses. Robyn Hitchcock's "Linctus House" reflects his experience of losing his close connection with his wife: "Couldn't stand to leave her side in the warm heat of love," … "now saying hello takes a lot of sweat" (Hitchcock, 1990, track 7). He conveys his reunification with his only sibling, his sister, by choosing the song … "My sister," and speaks about his cruelty to his sister, because he was "so afraid of the night" and "loved her" (Antony & the Johnsons, 2005, track 5). Arthur Lee sings about asking for help with his misery, and I think of Robert asking for my help. As I hear the last line of the song, "I always see your face," (Lee, 1969, track 10) I think about his increased capacity to take me in and hold the image of my face. Robert notices, "This is really helping me a lot, doing this with you." I find myself feeling more connected to Robert than I ever felt before. I feel myself "falling in love with the patient" (Meyer, 2000; Winnicott, 1949, 1969), in a way that a mother would feel when playing with her child, witnessing her child's developmental bursts. Music becomes a shared third (Ogden, 1994). Robert declares, "We now have our own little island."

I ask Robert to bring in photographs of his mother before she broke her back. I see a young, able-bodied mother holding her red-haired baby and smiling into the camera. That evening words from the song "How Could I Ever Know?" from the musical *The Secret Garden* (Norman & Schulman, 1992) come to mind. The singer asks for forgiveness for leaving and hope for a new way of loving "now that we are apart." While writing this chapter, I realize the story of *The Secret Garden* parallels our discovery of a shared interest in music. A child has lost his mother. The father's grief is so immense he withdraws from his son, who becomes sick and disabled. His feisty cousin comes to live with them, finding a secret garden, which has gone untouched since the mother's death. She brings the garden back to life, and the little boy is healed. I am the feisty cousin. Robert, the disabled child. Music is our secret garden.

We progress forward, with music as our anchor. I find my affection growing steadily for Robert as our work progresses. I think of the quote by Richard Fox, "While we should not speak of a 'cure by love' we should be equally cautious of a suggesting that there can be a cure without love," (1998, as cited in Meyer, 2000, p. 360).

Tears, not rage

Robert begins to bring more family photos to our sessions, as an entry point into his past. He talks about the impending marriage of one of his daughters. For the first time he shows me several photos of his mother when she was ill. She's propped up like a rag doll, her eyes are shut. In each picture my client's newborn children are laying in her lap, and she is incapable of holding them or seeing them. As Robert shares these photos, he begins to cry. "How I wish my mother could be here for this wedding. How I wish my mother could have been here to see my children grow." I say, "How I wish your mother could have been well enough to see you grow up." He begins to sob heartily now, speaking about a memory he hasn't had in 40 years, of a school project he did with his mother. He tells me how he loved that time with her, and longs for her. In certain moments between us, he feels like he did with his mother when she was healthy. Such moments are bittersweet. I say that after almost 12 years of treatment, he is finally allowing himself to grieve the loss of his mother.

> You lost your mother twice, once to her illness and another time when she died. You are grieving the loss of the healthy mother you once had. You are crying a lifetime full of tears. They were all stored up. Now they are here.

As I say this, his sobbing becomes harder. He uses up most of my tissues and apologizes for repeatedly blowing his nose. When I reference my young children, he says, "Now you have a two-year-old, a four-year-old, and a 50-year-old." This is the first time Robert ever cried with me.

Regression and tough love

After many years of substantial progress, Robert experiences a harrowing six-month regression after the death of his father and following an argument with his only son, which results in an estrangement between them. He becomes so decompensated, he takes disability leave time from work.

During this difficult treatment juncture, I have a dream: *I am in an underground music club with Robert, which is a cave-like setting, in his hometown. We are listening to a terrific punk rock band and having a great time together. Suddenly, everything shifts. I realize I am trapped and need to escape. I run out of the club, into the street, but I am barefoot, without a cell phone, and without my wallet. I have escaped, but with no way home.*

Like the dream, we shift suddenly from connection through music, into disconnection, and I desperately want to escape. This captures my attempts to stay afloat during that time: After many sessions of Robert spouting venomous words about his son and threatening to kill himself if he loses his leave time from work, I say something that startles us both: "This isn't therapy, this is a tirade!" He shouts back, "You are a tough-love therapist! Our therapy is coming to an end if I cannot speak the way I want to in here. I pay for this therapy. This is MY treatment!" Forcefully I state, "No, this is our treatment. There are two people in this room."

In subsequent sessions the tirades continue, particularly around his threat to kill himself (a parasuicidal threat) if he loses his leave time from work.

Despite my many attempts to intervene, his rages continue. Thinking of Nancy McWilliams' (2004) comment that the patient needs the therapist to be a worthy opponent, I say: "I am going to tell you something very important. Listen closely." He pauses to listen. I lay down a line:

> It is important to know that if you choose a path of self-destruction I can't support you. But I don't have the capacity to stop you. This treatment has been very hard work for both of us. I will continue to work with you and build on what we've done together, but I won't be a participant in your self-destruction.

He returns to his rage about his son. I stop him and say, "Were you able to hear what I just said?" With his head hanging, his body collapsing, I hear the voice of a small child, "That you won't support my self-destruction."

Following this exchange, multiple breakthroughs occur. He acknowledges with gratitude, "My life would be in shambles were it not for therapy." We have survived, yet again. Unlike the dream, we find our way back home.

From diseased wood emerges art

After finding our way home again, Robert brings me a gift of his woodturning for the first time. It is stunning. "The wood is very rare. It is red mulberry," he says. At the top part of the round container, the wood is jagged, uneven, and a dark rich brown. The lower part of the vase has swirls of light golden brown. At the bottom, there is a small jagged hole. There are slight punctures in the wood, which he explains are due to insects, but he feels they add to the beauty. I hold the vase with the care and tenderness with which I held my newborn daughters, clutching it close to my chest. I slide my hands down the sides that are rough, jagged, then smooth and curved. As I look inside I see a small card with a note, "Thank you for helping me through a tough time. Robert."

He explains to me for the first time the process of how he turns wood, from beginning to end. He goes on long journeys through the woods where the trees have grown chaotically. "I find distressed wood that is on its way to becoming dirt." He describes that the trees he finds have already collapsed and are usually diseased. "I give the trees a second life" and "hopefully a good long life." Without speaking the words, we both know that he is also speaking about our work and himself. I hold this vase, knowing our work is like the distressed wood it originated from. From disease and distress emerge a second life, and hopefully a good, long life.

The patient holds the therapist

In our sixteenth year of treatment, I endure a highly unexpected pregnancy, a traumatic and very dangerous miscarriage, which significantly impacts my physical health for an extended period of time. With considerable thought, concerned that he might assume the worst, I share with Robert that I suffered a miscarriage. I say I will need to reduce our session frequency to once a week for a while. As I speak, my voice begins to crack, and tears roll down my cheeks. In this moment, I am not the sturdy therapist he has known. I am shattered and vulnerable. Empathically, he directly looks at me and says, "I am sorry this happened to you. You have helped me so much. I don't need you in the way I did before. I am better now." For so many years, I held him. In this moment, he holds me.

The patient grows young again, the therapist grows up

Eighteen years into our therapy Robert strides in confidently having reclaimed his youthful, fit, and slender body. He dives in vigorously, naming his internal conflicts, his profound grief about the loss of his "angelic mother," his unresolved lifelong guilt, and his unfulfilled longings for greater closeness with his wife. As he begins to rant about his son, he holds up his hand like a crossing guard and says, "No I won't go there today, there's my id again! I know that doesn't help me."

Having moved from a disorganized, preoccupied, insecure attachment style, he now frequently demonstrates an earned-secure attachment style (Main, 1995). In the early years of our work, he had "no friends, just acquaintances" and led an impoverished life. Eighteen years later, he has a full, meaningful life. He has a close-knit group of friends, takes long walks with his dog, teaches woodturning, enjoys being an involved grandfather, attends a meet-up group he coordinates, listens to his vast music collection, and attends group and individual therapy. His relationship with his sister is repaired, and he visits her regularly. With a modest inheritance from his father, and a pension on the way, he is able to retire from his stressful job. He lives in a new home bathed with sunlight, with no garage to hide in, his beautiful woodturning creations on the shelves. He has left behind the garage where he would torture himself. When speaking of taking apart the furniture in his garage during his recent move, he stated,

> I had to take the garage apart myself. No one could do it for me. I have real happiness in my life, but I am also guilty and conflicted about it. I don't really know yet how to allow myself to live this way, but I am trying. It is a whole new way of living.

A couple of years ago, I had a dream about Robert kicking me in the back. The next day Robert told me about a life-threatening road rage incident he had, and described a full dissociative episode. I felt devastated, shocked, blindsided. Had our therapy really made the gains I believed it had? I have a fleeting feeling I want to throw him out as I did before. But I'm a different therapist, and he's a different patient. Together, we are a different pair. Demonstrating the principle of rupture and repair, we quickly understand and regain emotional stability and perspective.

Despite moving forward, Robert still carries his traumatized past, and we still have significant work to do. Quoting Jody Messler Davies (2005), "Lest you believe that I am telling you some kind of psychoanalytic fairy tale in the land of the impossible, let me assure you that (Robert) can still be extremely difficult," (p 802). Robert has yet to resolve his enraged feelings towards his son, from whom he remains estranged. He still smokes cannabis a minimal to moderate amount as if to say, "While I am better, don't forget how terribly I suffered, how I survived my suffering, and how I am STILL surviving my suffering."

Recently, Robert asked, "Am I the patient you have worked with the longest?" Hesitating, to take mental stock, I say, "yes." He's pleased and talks about how he transferred colleges six times, never completing more than a community college associate's degree, and switched jobs every two years. He stayed in his last job for 15 years, which coincided with our work. "You didn't drop out of therapy," I add. "You stuck with me and I stuck with you." He smiles, soaking up my words. "I needed every minute, every hour," he says tearing up. He describes how our work has changed over time, adding, "During some of our recent sessions I felt like we were just getting started."

Let me tell you about a recent reverie that I associate with Bion's concept of the "container" function (Bion, 1962), and Ogden's "maternal reverie" (Ogden, 1994). This is the image in my mind: *Robert and I sit in my office in a moment of utter stillness. My mind drifts to thinking about my two children, and I fantasize that Robert is my child too, my beloved and difficult child. With a fervent curiosity I ask myself, what internal and musical worlds might the two of us explore together? I hear the sound of Sixto Rodriguez melodies singing through my office, while the "rain drinks champagne" (Rodriguez, 1970, track 10) on my office window and the moon glistens in on us encircling us in a glow. We are a resilient pair.*

Discussion

I believe healing comes through the transformative experience of the therapeutic relationship. As Winnicott states, "There is no such thing as a baby" (Winnicott, 1960). There is the baby *and* the mother. In long-term relational treatment, there is no such thing as a patient. There is the patient *and* the therapist. Traditional psychoanalytic treatment focuses on one mind, the mind of the patient. Contemporary psychoanalytic practice, as reflected in my work with Robert, focuses on the patient's mind, the psychotherapist's mind, and our interactions and impact on each other.

It is no accident that this case is 18 years in the making. Robert began our work in an infantile, primitive state, steadily progressing and regressing through each stage of childhood and adolescent development, and finally into adulthood.

During my journey with Robert I have often questioned why I continued in treatment with such a relentlessly difficult patient. Was I a masochist? A martyr? A savior or saint? I know my own powerful motivations, both conscious and unconscious, were complex. When his vicious projections seemed intolerable, and my own countertransference responses unbearable, I cursed myself for sticking with it. I have cursed my mentor Judy who encouraged me to do so. As I write this, I am resolved. I see it was kismet. Without this patient, I wouldn't have grown into the therapist I was meant to become. And, he wouldn't have grown into the man he was meant to become.

Recently, Robert stated, "I am indebted to you for many reasons, I have fundamental insight into myself, now more than ever. It took me 18 years to come to this place. I appreciate you, you sent me on this journey." Melanie Klein (1957) stated, "One major derivative of love is the feeling of gratitude," (p. 187). It isn't just the patient who is grateful. Without Robert's fervent commitment to our treatment, I would not have been sent on this remarkable journey.

For an individual with severe developmental trauma to rework early attachment patterns and "grow young again" (Galassi, 1997) with a "good enough" psychotherapist (Winnicott, 1960), Robert's attachment with me allowed him to rework old patterns, resume stalled development, and change. Robert wasn't the only one of us to change. He gave me the chance to "grow up" as a psychotherapist as he "grew young again." And he gave me a chance to "grow young" again too. I recently recalled myself at ten and 11 writing fantastical stories, creating "timelessness that made me forget time" (Osbon, 1991). After a series of traumas in my adolescence, I stopped writing stories for 37 years. Robert allowed me to "grow young again" by giving me a story I knew I needed to write.

References

Antony and the Johnsons. (2005). "You are my sister" on *I am a bird now*. Bloomington, IN: Secretly Canadian.

Bion, W.R. (1962). *Learning from experience*. New York, NY: Rowman & Littlefield.

Bromberg, P. (1998). *Standing in the spaces*. New York, NY: Psychology Press.

Fox, R.P. (1998). The "unobjectionable positive" countertransference. *Journal of the American Psychoanalytic Association*, *46*, 1067–1087.

Fraiberg, S., Adelson, E. & Shapiro, V. (1975). Ghosts in the nursery: A psychoanalytic approach to the problems of impaired infant-mother relationships. *Journal of American Academy of Child Psychiatry*, *14*(3), 387–421.

Galassi, S. (1997). *Picasso's one liners*. New York, NY: Artisan.

Hitchcock, R. (1990). "Linctus house" on *Eye*. Minneapolis, MN: Twin Tone Records.

Klein, M. (1957). *Envy and gratitude*. New York, NY: Basic Books.

Kohut, H. (1971). *The analysis of the self: A systemic approach to the psychoanalytic treatment of narcissistic personality disorders*. New York, NY: International University Press.

Lee, A. (1969). "Always see your face" on *Love*. New York, NY: Elektra Records.

Loewald, H.W. (1960). On the therapeutic action of psycho-analysis. *The International Journal of Psychoanalysis, 41*, 16–33.

Main, M. (1995). Attachment: Overview, with implications for clinical work. In S. Goldberg, R. Muir & J. Kerr (Eds.), *Handbook of attachment: Theory, research, and clinical applications* (pp. 407–474). New York, NY: Guilford Press.

McWilliams, N. (2004). *Psychoanalytic psychotherapy*. New York, NY: Guilford Press.

Messler Davies, J. (2005). Transformations of desire and despair: Reflections on the termination process from a relational perspective. *Psychoanalytic Dialogues, 15*, 779–805.

Meyer, W.S. (2000). The psychoanalytic social worker/the social worker psychoanalyst: What shall be our message? *Clinical Social Work Journal, 28*, 355–367.

Mitchell, S. & Black, M. (1995). *Freud and beyond*. New York, NY: Basic Books.

Norman, M. (Writer) & Schulman, S. (Director). (1992). *The secret garden*. Live performance at St. James Theatre, New York, NY.

Ogden, T.H. (1994). The analytic third: Working with intersubjective clinical facts. *The International Journal of Psychoanalysis, 75*, 3–19.

Osbon, A. (1991). *Joseph Campbell companion: Reflections on the art of living*. New York, NY: Harper Perennial.

Rodriguez, S. (1970). "Cause" on *Coming from reality*. Los Angeles, CA: Sussex Records.

Schaefer, R. (2003). *Bad feelings*. New York, NY: Other Press.

Searles, H. (1979). *Countertransference and related subjects*. Madison, CT: International University Press.

Stern, D.B. (2015). *Relational freedom: Emergent properties of the interpersonal field*. New York, NY: Routledge.

Wallin, D. (2007). *Attachment in psychotherapy*. New York, NY: Guilford Press.

Winnicott, D.W. (1949). Hate in the counter-transference. *The International Journal of Psychoanalysis, 30*, 69–74.

Winnicott, D.W. (1960). The ordinary mother and her baby. CW 6:1:7. From: *What irks the ordinary mother and her baby?* Quigley, J. and Benzie, I. (producers). London: BBC Radio Broadcast.

Winnicott, D.W. (1969). The use of an object. *The International Journal of Psychoanalysis, 50*, 711–716.

Winnicott, D.W. (1971). *Playing and reality*. London: Tavistock Publications.

Chapter 9

Masks, walls and metaphors

Reflections on long-term treatment

Kathleen Fargione

When I think of long-term treatment, I think of development. When an adult comes for treatment, asking for help solving a current problem or dealing with overwhelming pain, I am interested in assessing the strength and integration of their psychic structure. From an object relations perspective, I wonder about their internal world and the nature of the internal objects they have introjected. When development has gone well, resulting in a well-integrated sense of self and an internal world with good-enough objects, creating a robust psychic structure, a person is more or less prepared for life's challenges. When development has gone poorly, a person is left with a psychic structure akin to Swiss cheese – it is full of holes, places where psychic structure has been supplemented by defensive bulwarks. The nature and number of these defensive systems indicate the work that lies ahead.

Patients with weak, crumbling or even absent psychic structure will need much longer treatment than those whose foundations are solid and mostly well functioning. When there is no secure foundation for psychic growth, when internal objects are weak or absent or cruel, treatment will involve strengthening and sometimes building, almost from scratch, a psychic foundation that can withstand the stresses that come in even an ordinary life.

It therefore behoves therapists to be familiar with developmental theory to better equip them to assess their patients' developmental history and the sturdiness of their psychic structures. Psychoanalytic theory offers various paradigms for understanding psychic development. Two that have been attractive to me are John Bowlby's attachment theory (Bowlby, 1988; Slade, 2004; Sroufe, 1986) and Wilfred Bion's theory of container/contained and alpha function (Bion, 1991/1962; Eaton, 2011; Riesenberg-Malcolm, 2001; Symington and Symington, 1996). Each of these theories lays out a paradigm for development. This chapter begins by giving a brief description of these theories and then offers two case studies to illustrate how each theory contributed to my understanding of the clinical material.

Theoretical background

Bowlby's attachment theory

Influenced by the ethologist Konrad Lorenz, John Bowlby (1988) recognized the evolutionary necessity for safety (both physical and psychic), and proposed that infants become deeply attached to their caregivers. Mary Ainsworth's research on infants in a "strange situation" showed that an infant accommodates his attachment needs to the personalities of his caregivers (Ainsworth, Blehar, Waters, and Wall, 1978). A secure infant learns that emotions can safely be shared and jointly understood, thus building the foundation for both affect regulation and mentalization (Fonagy, Gergely, Jurist, and Target, 2002). An insecure infant, on the other hand, learns that his emotions are not well attended to, either because they are not tolerated at all, or because the caregiver escalates rather than regulates them. The insecure infant either shuts off all of his emotions, relying exclusively on his rational mind, or is swamped by his emotions, eschewing thinking and relying on emotions to guide his behaviors (Slade, 2004). The first type of insecure infant would be called avoidant (avoiding feelings), and the second type called resistant/ambivalent (uncertain his feelings will be attended to by his caregivers). In an adult, these respective attachment styles would be called dismissing and preoccupied.

Another type of attachment – disorganized – has also been identified (Hesse and Main, 2000; Main and Solomon, 1990). In this style the infant has no organized strategy for maintaining proximity to his caregiver or for managing his own emotions. This happens most frequently when the infant's parents are frightening or frightened (often as a result of their own unresolved trauma).

Attachment research has continued to build on Bowlby's original insights, showing that behavior patterns developed in an infant's first relationships become internalized (Main, Kaplan, and Cassidy, 1985) and passed on to the next generation (Hesse, 1999).

Fonagy's mentalization

Peter Fonagy and his colleagues have provided a critical link in this intergenerational transmission of attachment styles through their concept of mentalization (Fonagy et al., 2002), and its extension, parental reflective functioning (Slade, 2005). Mentalization is the ability to reflect on ourselves and our feelings and also to keep others' feelings and opinions in mind. Slade (2005) has been able to show that a parent's ability to "reflect upon and hold the inner life of his child" (p. 270) is directly related to the child's development of a secure or an insecure or disorganized attachment. Fonagy's concept of mentalization thus brings attachment research full circle. Those with secure attachments where feelings are discussed openly develop a robust capacity for mentalization and, when they become parents, are able to keep in mind their child and his feelings, fostering a secure attachment in the next generation. Insecure and unresolved caregivers, on the other hand, have distorted, forgotten or remained overwhelmed by their own feelings and so find their child's feelings intolerable and painful. Thus, they turn away from or distort those needs as they have turned away from and distorted their own needs (Slade, 2000).

Bion's alpha function and containment

Wilfred Bion (1991/1962) used different terms to describe development. According to Bion, an infant initially is unable to tolerate certain amounts of distress (raw sensations, which Bion called beta elements) and looks to his caregiver to contain his distress and return it to him in more manageable form. This process Bion called the caregiver's alpha function. Through his parents' alpha function the infant takes back his now more manageable distress *and* develops his own alpha function. Distress is then able to be thought about, and this process of taking in and building his own alpha function creates for the infant a well-functioning mind capable of thinking rather than being emotionally overwhelmed (Riesenberg-Malcolm, 2001).

As the infant introjects the parents' alpha function, he gradually builds his own container where raw sensations (beta elements) can be metabolized. Unmetabolized beta elements cannot be used in thinking. They can only be evacuated – projected. When a parent holds and soothes a distressed baby, somehow, without understanding the words, the baby calms. Soon he may be able to do some soothing himself, remembering the voice or hands or rhythms of the parent. The baby is building his own container, his own alpha function.

Bion said that alpha elements gradually build up and make a "contact barrier" (1991/1962) that demarcates the conscious from the unconscious mind. A patient without a contact barrier, or with a very leaky one, will not be able to distinguish internal from external reality, or conscious from unconscious thoughts, or hallucinations from dreams, or dreams from memories. Hallucinations seem vibrant and alive; dreams seem like actual events. Physical reality seems pale compared to these overwhelming psychic experiences. Bion said that treatment is the repair of communication between the conscious and the unconscious mind. This idea has intrigued me and was particularly helpful in working with Suzanne.

Object relations theory

Awareness of object relations runs like a thread through all of my work. Anne Alvarez (1977, 1992, 2012) has influenced my thinking about object relations and long-term treatment. Writing about her work with abused and damaged children, Alvarez describes internal worlds filled with vindictive, intimidating, frightening objects. She points to Bion's emphasis on the importance of a containing object and reminds us that some objects can "provide inadequate containment" (2012, p. 58). Bion's container/contained theory made room in Kleinian theory "for a theory of deficit" (2012, p. 58). Many moments in my two clinical examples made me think of deficit and the importance of becoming a containing object.

Trauma theory

Through the work of Bessel van der Kolk (2005) and Bruce Perry (1995), among others, we now know a great deal about the sequelae of early relational trauma. The work of both men has alerted us to the damage that early trauma wreaks on a developing psyche. Trauma creates neurological and endocrinological changes, and unintegrated, fragmented memories, interfering with the formation of a cohesive sense of self. More importantly, early trauma precludes normal development, so that healing requires catching up on the psychic growth that should have been happening while the trauma was occurring. Individuals who have suffered early, relational trauma from their caregivers have deep and easily reopened cracks in their psychic foundations. Safety must be instituted and must begin in the patient's own body before other work can take place. The patient must develop the capacity to regulate their physiological responses so that ordinary life does not trigger hyper- or hypoarousal. I am not trained in this kind of body work. When needed, I collaborate with a therapist trained in sensorimotor psychotherapy as developed by Pat Ogden (Ogden, Minton, and Pain, 2006) and Peter Levine (1997).

Case examples

In this chapter I will discuss two long-term treatments, each from a predominantly different perspective. The first patient, whom I will call Martha, presented with an avoidant or dismissing attachment style. She had all the earmarks of this style of attachment; she valued autonomy over intimacy, she built walls rather than bridges, and she eschewed her feelings and distanced herself from any comfort relationships might offer. The second patient, whom I will call Suzanne, was far more fragile than Martha. She had experienced early relational trauma, relied heavily on dissociation and had developed little alpha function. Her conscious and unconscious thoughts were a muddle. Her dreams, memories and hallucinations were indistinguishable.

Martha

I met Martha when I was working in a day treatment program for emotionally disturbed adolescents. Our worked spanned 16 years. She and her husband David began working with me to address some of the tangles in their relationship with their son who was in our program. Both Martha and David appeared extremely reluctant to come in for family sessions. This was something that was encouraged in our program, if only to offer parents the support they needed in raising a challenging child. Initially, it was only Martha who was willing to come, as David had strong fears that therapy might do more harm than good. By the time David was on board, Martha and I had begun a conversation that needed finishing. With David's consent, we continued our work, concomitant with our couples' work. So it happened that I had two appointments with this family each week, one with Martha alone, and one with both Martha and David. I realize that this was a rather unorthodox approach, but somehow it worked. One reason I think it worked is that David was never jealous of my work with Martha, only grateful that someone wanted to understand his wife and then help him understand her – and himself.

Although the story of my work with Martha and David as a couple is a compelling one, in this chapter I will be focusing on my work with Martha, with only occasional references to the couples' work as they illustrate the progress Martha was making. Nor will I be discussing my work with their son or the impact of his struggles on his younger brother, which is another whole story in itself. In the course of our work, both Martha and David grew enormously in their abilities to understand themselves, and then one another, and then their son and his brother.

Our early work was often about family disagreements. Neither Martha nor David felt heard or respected by one another, and they never resolved their disagreements. Each seemed to have the idea that a discussion meant trying to "win" an argument. We worked at reframing this, trying to imagine discussions that were exercises in curiosity about what the other was thinking and feeling. I asked them once when they had last asked their partner how he or she felt about something. They each looked completely taken by surprise by my query and said, immediately, that neither had *ever*, in 14 years of marriage, asked their partner this question.

Martha worked hard at protecting herself from feelings. I believed that if she could talk about some of these feelings she would feel better, and she did – but the "feeling better" took many years. What came first was feeling much, much worse. All of her inability to trust others or to find comfort in relationships was brought into the transference. When I asked if she had thought about our last conversation she would answer that she tried very hard *not to*. She told me that even driving over to our appointment she would turn up the music as loud as she could, trying to drown out any thoughts or accompanying feelings. For many years, I carried the thread of our conversation from session to session.

First trust

Within months of our first meeting, Martha told me that she had once left David. This had happened years ago, early in their marriage, but the feelings were still raw and unmetabolized. She couldn't remember how long she had been gone (anywhere from one to six weeks) and she had virtually no memory of her thoughts and feelings at the time beyond the fact that she had not been happy. She was not able to tell me what had made her return, only that things had been better for a little while, but then reverted to the tension-filled distance that marked so much of their relationship. I asked if she could remember when the tension had returned, and she answered with a specific date, 11 years before. I asked what had happened on that date and she said she had had a miscarriage, "I was terribly sad and really angry." And she and David had *never* talked about this.

Martha took an enormous risk in telling me this. There was an obvious desire for healing, but this was accompanied by an equally strong fear about how I would react – that I would judge her in some way. She herself noted that she kept moving her chair back, through the wall, if possible, to restore the distance between us that her revelation had shortened. Martha paid a huge price for telling me this painful piece of her history. It was not only my reaction that she feared, it was bearing the feelings that would accompany bringing forth these memories. When I asked the following week how she was, she said, "I felt the worst I have ever felt in my life."

Avoidant attachments and defenses

Initially, I found it confusing that Martha felt worse, rather than better, after unburdening herself. I had forgotten that defenses are always there for a reason. Soon enough I learned the powerful back story to her fears of allowing me to know her in a more intimate way. She told me that as a four-year-old she had burned her hand on the stove. Attempting to see what her mother was cooking, she had placed her hand on a burner and hoisted herself up, not realizing that the burner was very hot. I winced hearing this story and had a vision of a crying child and an alarmed and comforting mother. My vision was all wrong. Martha, already well practiced in avoidant attachment, had not cried, but had gone to the living room and held her hand, fearing her mother's reprimand more than the pain of the burn. In fact her mother had not reprimanded her, and had bandaged her hand, but the critical piece of the story is Martha's fear and her inability to assume that she would be comforted. She brought these same expectations to her relationship with me – she could not imagine that sharing these memories could be comforting.

I made the mistake of assuming that finding someplace where she could be vulnerable would be a relief to Martha. She quickly corrected that notion; for her, being vulnerable meant she could be hurt. What she had shared with me could be used against her.

At the beginning of our work, Martha had told me that she had had a "normal" childhood, growing up in a two-parent family in a suburban neighborhood. What she didn't say, and what she could not have known, was that she had come to believe that her deepest needs for recognition and affirmation would seldom be met. Her parents provided food, clothing, shelter, education. They took care of her and her siblings when they were sick. They were "good parents." What her parents did not provide was space for holding and thinking about feelings, probably because it was not something that either of them had experienced themselves. Uncomfortable with their own feelings, they had offered no safe place for their children's feelings to be explored and understood.

Martha had an armamentarium of defenses against experiencing her feelings. She built walls. Once, when I was rejoicing that a few bricks in the wall were down, she told me,

> There are two walls – one to keep feelings from everyone else and one to keep them from me. Feelings are not good things. In my family the times emotions were expressed were ugly. I can't let the wall down. Then I'll be vulnerable and get hurt.

We see here a compartmentalized mind. Such a mind has a terrible time trying to make sense of life; that would require understanding feelings, and those were safely locked away. "My feelings," Martha told me,

> I have to lock them in a box. There are only two ways to handle feelings, keep them locked up or carry them around and hit everyone with them. I feel like there are two roads and you're telling me to go down a third – but I don't know where I am going or what it will be like when I get there and I don't have any headlights.

Before Martha got to a better place she would have to have a relationship with me that was strong enough to be a "remedy for her fear" as she explored her feelings. This is, I believe, part of the reason that long-term relational work with a consistent therapist is so important. Martha had a very good mind, but it was strong in thinking and defended against feelings, and we had to build in her the capacity to tolerate and explore her feelings. In other words, we were building psychic structure – the structure that had not been built in her as a child. The more open she was, the more it hurt. At times, the trust she was building with me would fall apart.

What I was asking was scary and often overwhelmed her. Once she wrote me a note that said: "Am I too old to run away from home?" Ten days later she ran away from me, cancelling all our appointments. This was about 18 months into treatment. She wrote to me and explained what was happening to her as she shared more with me:

> I don't feel that I am a good therapy participant because everywhere I turn, I put up more walls. Sometimes you ask me things that are such foreign concepts. Every time I think about it, I am overwhelmed by the emotions I have. Once the wall started coming down there was no retreat and no escape. If I consider them at all, the emotions overpower me. I feel like I am drowning. The wall is there to protect me and it can't do that once it's down, and if I try to acknowledge the emotions, I just relive them. I can't control them and I can't make them stop. I would like to be able to know what I feel and not be afraid of what I feel. I would like to fully love my family and to teach my children how to love and not to be afraid. I would like to be able to trust in the love and not let the fear beat that down.

And so we began again to build trust, to banish fear. This pattern repeated many times – the fear, the quitting, the returning, the work, the fear …

She said that talking about her life was like throwing a drowning person a rock, and trying to find her feelings was like searching America for elephants. I suggested that she might have to *feel* the feelings before she could know them or name them or understand them. She said "the animal out in the fog just ate me! *That* is not a good plan! *That* is a *stupid-ass* idea." I asked her if understanding her feelings was really worse than the way she currently was feeling and she replied, "It's like jumping into a typhoon! There's no way to protect yourself!"

Learning to cry

The worst outcome of telling me something painful was for her to cry. This was nearly intolerable. The first time it happened I commented that she was crying – that her affect matched her story – and she was upset with me for "announcing" it. She said, "*I* don't want to know that I am crying. I don't want to be around *myself* when I am crying. And I certainly don't want *you* to see me crying *and comment on it*!"

But there were deeper fears than fears of being ridiculed or of me seeing her cry. Four and a half years into our journey we had a significant conversation. David had verbally attacked her and criticized her parenting and had not apologized. I commented that when she is hurt she puts up the walls again. She said "I need them. It is not like I want them up – it just happens, it just is." What follows is a small piece of our conversation that day:

K: I have an idea. When you put the walls up, it is not just protective; it is to hold you together because you are afraid of falling apart. Does this make any sense to you?

M: It is exactly how I feel. I never wanted you to know. I do not like your saying it. It makes it too real.

K: It is real already. It is there – saying it helps us understand it. You are afraid of shattering. You are afraid that you will break like a china doll.

M: I do not like that. I am afraid of coming apart and never being able to be put together again, like a shattered mirror. Once broken, I could never be repaired.

Here we see again how necessary her defenses were – they held her together. The fear of shattering was overwhelming. Dismantling these defenses had to be done with great care and with the belief that she was now strong enough to hold herself together from the inside out.

Later, she asked me,

M: How did you know that I felt that I might fall apart?

K: I could see it. I could feel it. It was right in front of me.

M: I knew it, but I didn't know it. My mind was telling it to me, but I didn't believe it. When you said it, it was true. It wasn't true until you said it. I don't like that you know that about me. How do you know that I won't break?

K: You are stronger than you think. You think that all your strength is in that shield but it is inside you too.

We see here that we were building psychic structure. Every step was tentative. Every new achievement was precarious.

Enlarging the window of tolerance

Treatment for patients like Martha, who have an insecure attachment and are easily swamped by their feelings, must include an enlarging of their capacity to tolerate feelings. Pat Ogden (Ogden, Minton, and Pain (2006) calls this capacity "the window of tolerance" (pp. 26–40). Some days the window opened a crack, other times it was sealed shut. Gradually, it opened more and more and was able to stay open even in the face of distressing feelings – but that was years in coming. In the end, Martha told me that all of treatment was about learning to trust me. Our relationship, I think, is what gave her a secure base on which to build a less defended sense of herself.

She gradually developed the capacity to talk about her distress and to tolerate the feelings which accompanied this. She often "practiced" talking about something difficult with me and then tried to have that same conversation with David and me together. She talked about her miscarriage with me, and then with David. Together, they mourned the child they had lost and the years that they missed when they could not communicate. They found one another again. Martha began to take comfort in David's presence. She told me, "He takes the place of the walls" (a concept straight from attachment theory)! They learned about one another's shortcomings and were able to understand one another in new ways. Martha learned that David's hesitations were from his own fears rather than a lack of commitment to her. David learned that Martha had a thin skin, something he had never before imagined. They rediscovered their love and respect for one another. She learned to let David tease her. They laughed together.

Suzanne

Suzanne's treatment was very different from Martha's. Unlike Martha, Suzanne had endured early, prolonged relational trauma. This had left her with profound holes in her psychic development which required long treatment.

Suzanne was 20 years old when I first met her. We worked together for ten years. She had a conviction (but no actual memories) that she had been sexually abused at a very early age. She had terrifying images of being tied up, of being threatened with knives, of being raped. She had pains in her body which had no physical explanations. She cut. She dissociated frequently. As a child, she had wet the bed. As an adult, she had horrifying nightmares. She brought a doll to therapy. She was haunted by suicidal thoughts. She saw nooses hanging from her ceiling. Twice she admitted herself to the hospital in order to keep herself safe. After the first few years of treatment, the suicidal thoughts and the cutting stopped. She began bringing a dog to therapy rather than her favorite doll. In an effort to address her physiological distress she began working with a therapist trained in sensorimotor psychotherapy once a week in addition to her weekly appointment with me.

I could see that Suzanne's psychic balance was precarious. I felt that a small breeze might blow her over, like the fork that one can balance ever so carefully on a toothpick on the edge of a glass. One touch, one unexpected word and all might fall to pieces.

Somehow she had gotten through her horrific childhood. She had compartmentalized her mind – one part kept all of her secrets, one part went to school. Amazingly, she learned. When she could not allow herself to know her own story, she wrote stories of other children, homeless children lost and estranged from their families, little girls with no underwear.

In the second year of our work she showed me a story she had written about a young woman who had been raped, but something good had come of the rape, she had become pregnant with three little girls. Suzanne told me that she thought there were parts of herself that she had always hoped would grow, but she feared had died. Now, she realized that she had had those little girls, but they had needed to stay hidden inside her. Now, she said, they can come out. We talked about all the ways that she, now an adult woman, could care for those little girls, the fragmented little Suzanne. We worked in metaphor, first making a safe place for the child who had been so frightened.

Nightmares

Suzanne's nightmares woke her in the middle of the night; she would be drenched in sweat, teeth clamped tightly on her mouth guard, heart beating furiously. She reminded me of the children examined by Bruce Perry (2006) after they were rescued from the Branch Davidian compound in Waco, Texas (pp. 57–80). Their resting heart rate was between 100 and 170 beats/minute (normal range is significantly lower).

Suzanne described her nightmares as "haunting." She dreamt that her father was working in a building that was crumbling. She dreamt she was getting married and her mother was putting on her veil, but the flowers were all dead. She dreamt that her parents abducted her and kept her locked in a shed. She dreamt that everyone in her family was killed by the police, but it was she who was covered in blood. She dreamt her father had a dollhouse on a bed of poison sand that he was trying to give to her. She dreamt about lambs that turned into tigers. She dreamt about combing her hair with a butcher knife. She dreamt she was in a house and she knew that something bad was going on. Upstairs she found two little girls and an infant boy who had been either neglected or abused. They were all crying. Every week, there were more dreams, unspooling one after the other into the space between us.

I believe these dreams were Suzanne's attempts to make sense of her childhood experiences. She had never been able to adequately metabolize her early experiences; no one had helped her to contain and transform them. Bion's (1991/1962) theory of alpha function gave me a way to think about Suzanne. She had had virtually no chance to develop alpha function. Not only were her parents at times terrifying, even in the ordinary course of daily life they were angry and unattuned. They did not offer her their own alpha function (perhaps because their own were so stunted). I was encountering what Symington and Symington (1996) described as "either the absence of a container or a container that is damaged or porous and not able to hold the contained, like a muslin bag trying to hold water" (p. 55). Suzanne's terrors came leaking out in her nightmares.

Suzanne seldom brought events from her day-to-day life for us to discuss. Mostly, she brought dreams – current dreams which often triggered memories of past dreams. It was as if these dreams were more real than what was happening or had happened in her day-to-day life. I realized that these dreams *were* the stuff of her life. These dreams were her constant psychic companions, fragments of her unsuccessful efforts to metabolize her early traumatic experiences. She told me once that she had been realizing that as a child she was more awake when she was asleep and more asleep when she was awake – that her dreams were more real than her life.

Sometimes the things Suzanne told me left me uncertain about whether I was hearing a dream, a hallucination or an actual event. Within our first year of meeting Suzanne told me that she had been raped by the devil when she was in high school. She described the scene in her bedroom and she was quite clear that it had been the devil who had raped her. I listened and drew her attention to the emotions accompanying this memory. I did not know if it was a nightmare or a hallucination. Years later, without our ever returning to talk about this, Suzanne told me that she realized that it had been her father who had raped or abused her. I commented that at the time it must have seemed as if only a demon could do such a thing.

Building alpha function

Suzanne's mind was a muddle of unmetabolized experiences. Primary processes and some rudimentary secondary processes were all mixed together. Her conscious mind was not demarcated from her unconscious mind – unconscious fears, anxieties, and fragments of memories were all present. Symington and Symington (1996), writing about situations where there is missing or inadequate alpha function, said, "there is no separation of the mental phenomena into conscious and unconscious functions and consequently the material seems confused and often resembles a dream or a hallucination" (p. 65).

We talked about some of her dreams many times and, as she developed more alpha function, her understanding of them grew. She told me a dream that she had had when she was five or six. She said in the dream her parents were hurting her, but then she thought that they were not really her parents, they were two people dressed as garbage cans made to look like her parents. She said she realized that as a child she could not admit what her parents were doing, so her dream made it seem that it was "garbage people" hurting her.

Little by little, she grew stronger and her nightmares reflected this. About five years into treatment she said she had a nightmare where she was in her apartment and her parents were trying to break in. She said a friend was there and told her to go hide. She said, "No! I am going to call the police and I am going to go outside and tell them to stop bothering me." I asked her to compare her strength vis-à-vis her parents when she first left home to now. She said when she first left home, in her mind her parents looked like enormous monsters. Now, she said, they are still monsters, but they look old and weak and fragile.

Integration

One of the primary goals of therapy was, of course, integration. We wanted to integrate the fragmented memories of the past. We wanted to make a story about her life that Suzanne could live with. Suzanne began to "see" a little girl, dressed entirely in black, who came to visit her in her bedroom. She said she always thought the little girl was herself. She said in some ways the little girl frightened her because she knew that the girl knew something that she herself did not know. I talked about how she had dissociated when she was very young, giving all her bad memories to this little girl, and how necessary that had been to her survival. One part of her succeeded at school, the other was afraid at home. She kept the two separate. Now this little girl was coming to her, allowing her to become more integrated.

Six years into treatment, Suzanne told me:

> I had a dream a few nights ago, and the premise of the dream was that the little girl I was, died. She was murdered. But the me who is 26, is still alive. The little, lost ghost of the girl I once was, is with me, haunting me, though she doesn't mean to haunt me. It's just that she's so young, three or four years old, and the only way she knows how to communicate is by speaking to me through dreams. But those dreams translate into nightmares because the things she knows are too gruesome. But year by year, little by little, she and I are growing stronger. She is able to reveal to me the scary things of my past that I cannot remember, and I am able to hold the nightmares for her, as best I can, because I know, for the first time in my life, I am in a safe place. We are integrating, she and I, and setting ourselves free.

Integration brought its own fears. Several years later, when the little girl was still appearing to Suzanne, she said she could remember the little girl going places with her when she was a child and then she would not be so afraid. I said the little girl saved her life, because the little girl was a part of herself that carried all her fears so that she could go to school and live as normally as possible. I said, "now the little girl is going to grow up too." Suzanne teared up and said she doesn't want the little girl to grow up because then she will be alone again. I think she felt that she would have no one to help her carry her fears, no container. A month later, Suzanne said that she had been looking around her apartment and seeing it with new eyes, realizing that it looked like a little girl lives there. She said she had had to make it that way, to make it safe for the little girl.

In the last two years of our work, before I retired, Suzanne's dreams began to change. Although she still had many terrifying dreams, she began having other dreams with other feelings. She dreamt she saw her father and was angry with him, yelling at him and confronting him, saying "you abused me when I was just a little girl!" When she did have a bad dream she was more likely to respond with anger than with fear. She dreamt she went shopping and saw her parents and felt rage rather than fear. She told me she remembered reading that it is common for those who have experienced incest to feel rage. Suzanne said that this rage was a new feeling. She said as a child she had not felt rage, rather she felt she had been wearing a mask, pretending to be normal.

Suzanne found therapy exhausting and terrifying. But she brought a determination to it. She did not want the trauma to win. She did not want her parents to win. She told me once that her life was like beginning to watch a movie in the middle where you are never going to know the first part of the movie. I said she may never know the first part of the movie, but she has learned that she can be both writer and director of the second half of the movie. One night as she was falling asleep she felt something warm and wonderful all through her body. She said she realized that it was healing.

Reflections

Both Martha and Suzanne needed long-term treatment to rebuild the missing pieces in their psychic structures, to repair their internal damaged objects. Writing about them, I am struck by their similarities despite their profound differences. I find myself using some of the same words to describe them: compartmentalized, dissociated, fragile. What was different was the *degree* of their brokenness. Both patients dissociated, but Suzanne's dissociation was much more severe – whole pieces of herself and her memories had been dissociated. Martha feared fragmentation but was held together by her defenses, while Suzanne had almost no way to hold herself together other than dissociation or self-harm. Suzanne's very sense of herself was fragmented, with one little girl part of herself traumatized and holding her secrets, and another part of herself, shielded from the trauma, continuing to live a superficially normal childhood. When the reality of her trauma broke through her false "normalcy," she felt she was falling apart and she sought treatment. Martha had more ego strengths, but when her defenses no longer worked, when her anxieties began to threaten her psychic balance, she too, came for treatment.

Each woman needed to integrate parts of herself that had been locked away or dissociated. Integration for Martha began with learning to trust the relationship she had with me, learning that she could tell me things that would not be used against her. Her internal world changed. The ridiculing and critical internal objects got smaller and less powerful. She became more compassionate towards herself and David and their children. Her state of mind with regard to attachment went from dismissing to secure/autonomous. Defensive habits of flight or wall-building changed. She no longer worried that she would shatter. Her window of tolerance grew larger. She could take comfort in relationships.

Suzanne was far more damaged when we began our work. She had many moments of psychosis in her hallucinations and nightmares and dissociation. She had a precarious hold on her own mind, which had been traumatized when she was very young with no one to help her contain the trauma. In treatment I provided some alpha function to help her sort out and make sense of her early raw experiences. Slowly, she built the beginnings of alpha function and a container where neither had been before. She was able to acknowledge the horrors of her childhood without resorting to writing stories about other children. She felt stronger and more integrated. She took back into herself the little girl part of herself who had carried all her secrets. Her internal world, which had been filled with cruel, frightening objects and a terrified little girl self, began to make room for a self that could be righteously angry and cautiously hopeful. Most importantly, she began to find joy in life, telling me that one morning she had found herself saying "Joie de vivre," something she had learned years ago in her French class.

Such reconstructive work does not happen quickly. Healing takes time, time to build a sense of safety, time to reclaim one's body from trigger-quick hypo- or hyperarousal, time to integrate, time to reflect, time to grieve over all that has been lost or missed, time to introject good objects, time to build up a sense of a self capable of joy and empathy and agency. The fact that both Martha and Suzanne changed in substantive ways in all of these areas is a testament to their courage and their willingness to engage with me in difficult, often painful work over a long period of time.

References

Ainsworth, M. D. S., Blehar, M., Waters, E., & Wall, S. (1978). *Patterns of attachment.* Hillsdale, NJ: Lawrence Erlbaum Associates.

Alvarez, A. (1977). Problems of dependence and development in an excessively passive autistic boy. *Journal of Child Psychotherapy, 4*, 25–46.

Alvarez, A. (1992). *Live company: Psychoanalytic psychotherapy with autistic, borderline, deprived and abused children.* New York, NY: Brunner-Routledge.

Alvarez, A. (2012). *The thinking heart: Three levels of psychoanalytic therapy with disturbed children.* New York, NY: Routledge.

Bion, W. R. (1991/1962). *Learning from experience.* London: Karnac.

Bowlby, J. (1988). Developmental psychiatry comes of age. *The American Journal of Psychiatry, 145*, 1–10.

Eaton, J. (2011). *A fruitful harvest: Essays after Bion.* New York, NY: Basic Books.

Fonagy, P., Gergely, G., Jurist, E., & Target, M. (2002). *Affect regulation, mentalization and the development of the self.* New York, NY: Other Press.

Hesse, E. (1999). The adult attachment interview: Historical and current perspectives. In J. Cassidy & P. R. Shaver (Eds.), *Handbook of attachment: Theory, research, and clinical applications* (pp. 395–433). New York, NY: Guilford Press.

Hesse, E. & Main, M. (2000). Disorganized infant, child and adult attachment: Collapse in behavioral and attentional strategies. *Journal of the American Psychoanalytic Association*, *48*, 1097–1127.

Levine, P. (1997). *Waking the tiger: Healing trauma*. Berkeley, CA: North Atlantic Books.

Main, M. & Solomon, J. (1990). Procedures for identifying infants as disorganized/disoriented during the Ainsworth Strange Situation. In M. T. Greenberg, D. Cicchetti, & E. M. Cummings (Eds.), *The John D. and Catherine T. MacArthur Foundation series on mental health and development: Attachment in the preschool years: Theory, research, and intervention* (pp. 121–160). Chicago, IL: University of Chicago Press.

Main, M., Kaplan, N., & Cassidy, J. (1985). Security in infancy, childhood, and adulthood: A move to the level or representation. In I. Bretherton & E. Waters (Eds.), *Growing points of attachment theory and research*, Monographs of the society for research in child development, Vol. 50 (1–2), Serial No. 209 (pp. 66–194). Chicago, IL: University of Chicago Press.

Ogden, P., Minton, K., & Pain, C. (2006). *Trauma and the body: A sensorimotor approach to psychotherapy*. New York, NY: W. W. Norton & Co.

Perry, B. (1995). Childhood trauma, the neurobiology of adaptation, and "use-dependent" development of the brain: How states become traits. *Infant Mental Health Journal*, *16*(4), 271–289.

Perry, B. (2006). *The boy who was raised as a dog*. New York, NY: Basic Books.

Riesenberg-Malcolm, R. (2001). Bion's theory of containment. In C. Bronstein (Ed.), *Kleinian theory: A contemporary perspective* (pp. 164–171). Philadelphia, PA: Whurr.

Slade, A. (2000). The development and organization of attachment: Implications for psychoanalysis. *Journal of the American Psychoanalytic Association*, *48*, 1147–1174.

Slade, A. (2004). Two therapies: Attachment organization and the clinical process. In L. Atkinson & S. Goldberg (Eds.), *Attachment issues in psychopathology and intervention* (pp. 181–206). Mahwah, NJ: Lawrence Erlbaum Associates.

Slade, A. (2005). Parental reflective functioning: An introduction. *Attachment and Human Development*, *7*(3), 269–281.

Sroufe, L. A. (1986). Bowlby's contribution to psychoanalytic theory and developmental psychopathology. *Journal of Child Psychology and Psychiatry*, *27*, 841–849.

Symington, J. & Symington, N. (1996). *The clinical thinking of Wilfred Bion*. New York, NY: Brunner-Routledge.

van der Kolk, B. (2005). Developmental trauma disorder: Towards a rational diagnosis for children with complex trauma histories. *Psychiatric Annals*, *5*(5), 401–408.

Part III

How could it be otherwise?

Chapter 10

Being still

Sitting with suffering in long-term relational practice

Joan Berzoff

As relational practitioners, we are tasked with sitting with suffering. Our clients come to us with profound losses, betrayal, abuse, and violations to their basic integrity and well-being. Sometimes they come with terminal illnesses and are facing their impending deaths or the deaths of those around them. Many clients do not have words for their suffering.

When we sit with those who suffer in long-term treatment, we need to feel what they feel in our bones. We need to be willing to share what has felt too difficult to bear alone. We need to be present. We do not change suffering. We witness it. We experience it. Sometimes we can help to hold it. By holding it, we can help our clients to bear it. We give it words. In this way we also help to make suffering thinkable. To suffering, we bring our own passion and compassion. This is hard work. The very act of bearing suffering with another over the long-term changes not only the person who suffers, but sometimes the practitioner as well. This chapter muses on what it means to sit with suffering in long-term psychodynamic practice.

Client # 1

My client is a 49-year-old black engineer born in Soweto, South Africa. He is a very handsome and elegant man who was raised in crushing poverty, sharing a room with his mother and many cousins while he slept on the floor. His mother was 15 when he was born. His father has never been a part of his life.

His mother, who was uneducated and unemployed, beat him regularly and burned him with cigarettes. The scars are evident on his arms, his hands and his face. He describes his hunger, anger, poverty and helplessness as a child. Those feelings accompany him now as they did then. As a child, there was no legal or familial protection from child abuse, hunger or racism. As an adult, the only protection he derives from his suffering is to withdraw into movies and into surfing the internet.

He has come to me precisely because he feels himself to be "too cut off." The Latin American woman with whom he lives wants to marry him, but he is too shut down. He recognizes that their partnership will not last anyway. He does not love her. He says he is too damaged to love or be loved.

My client left South Africa at 17 and moved to London where he lived on couches, and then to the US, where he attended night school and then engineering school. He made a significant suicide attempt while in college and was hospitalized for a year. He later married a light-skinned Nigerian woman from a highly religious Pentecostal family hoping to gain acceptance into her family. She was repeatedly violent towards him and she ultimately divorced him. Parental alienation soon followed, and he rarely saw his three daughters as they grew up. After the divorce, he was shunned by her extended family. He is a very dark-skinned man. A part of his suffering he ascribes to the repeated racism he experiences at work and in his family, based on skin color. There is a passivity and an enduring helplessness to his suffering.

In his work, he eschews his colleagues. At home, he watches films online, losing himself in the computer while his girlfriend reads on the floor above. His suffering is immense and unending. He feels worthless and alone. He weeps inconsolably, given the deprivation and emotional poverty with which he lives and has lived. I feel desolate in sitting with him. We are awash in suffering: his, mine, ours. Given the immensity of his unalleviated and unbounded suffering, it is no wonder that his partner needs to go to another floor. I, too, wish that I could sometimes go somewhere else. Like him, however, I have no other room to go to. We face each other week after week in the same room at the same time.

We have been together for four years. I expect we will be together many more. It is not easy to be with someone so shut down. While a large part of me wants to accompany him in his suffering, (even if the years stretch interminably ahead), I also dread feeling too much sorrow, or its opposite, the deadness that he often carries to ward off the pain.

Client # 2

My next client of the day is a Palestinian woman who is 44. Tall, lithe, athletic, she rides her bike to every session, even in the dead of a snowy New England winter. I have seen her for five years. Her father was in prison for 20 years for political reasons; his prison terms occurred throughout her childhood. Her mother's marriage, arranged, was never satisfying. During her father's incarceration, her mother lived a highly controlled life, kept a virtual captive by her father's brother to whom she was subservient.

Growing up, my client suffered the demolition of their home at age 10, the loss of a grandparent who was killed when the Israeli army entered their home and fired on him, and the brief kidnapping of her sister when her sister was 12 and she was 14. Her elementary and secondary schools were open and shut capriciously. She was aware of her mother's subservient role and those of women in her community. At 18, she was able to leave the country to study abroad and did not return. A strong and articulate woman, she attracted a mentor who helped her get full aid for college and she did not return to Palestine.

My client became an elementary school teacher and gave birth to a female child. That child, now an adolescent, recently reported that there had been years of sexual abuse by a neighbor who was entrusted with her care while my client went to school. As my client could not protect her sister, mother, father or grandparents, she is wracked with anguish over not having been able to protect her child either. Most recently, she applied for citizenship and was turned down. She has to return to Palestine. Her daughter, who was born in the US, can stay. She curls into a ball in my office and wails. We are awash in her helplessness, her anger, her suffering and mine for her. The amount of grief, for her family members, her daughter and herself feels enormous and, at times, uncontainable.

Two clients, two people who suffer not only from poverty, racism, disenfranchisement, but from interpersonal traumas as well, bring seemingly unbearable pain to the session. With them, I suffer too. How do we bear suffering from a relational perspective?

Theories of suffering

There is a school of thought, and philosophical stance, that the relief of suffering is the ethical duty and the obligation of the practitioner. According to Levinas (1988), a philosopher who wrote about suffering, we are called upon to respond to others in need. We are called on to be hospitable to the other and to the other's suffering. This is an ethical calling and Levinas calls it the very basis for empathy. The other's cry for help, he suggests, demands a relational response. But paradoxically, he adds, we cannot ever fully know the other. While suffering appears relational, it always involves the person who is suffering and the one who responds. There is still a "self" and an "other" and a distance between them. But is there always such distance? Or must the practitioner find herself awash in the suffering of the other?

For Freud and for many others, there is something almost heroic in suffering. Freud viewed suffering as necessary for insight and change, like surgery without an anesthetic (Davies, 2011). Arthur Frank (1995) wrote that to be able to suffer is to be able to fully see. Henri Nouwen (1979), who coined the term the "wounded healer," reframed the sufferer from being a victim, to the sufferer being an actor, one who can master her suffering by ultimately overcoming it.

In almost all religions suffering has a larger purpose and it is part of a greater plan (Wilt, Exline, Lindberg, Park, and Pargament, 2017). In Judaism, God continually tests Job by inflicting indignities to his body and soul. Job maintains his faith in spite of his suffering (Job, *The New King James Version*). In Christianity, suffering is seen as ennobling and even redemptive (Green and Palpant, 2014, p. 263). As Christ suffered, so did his disciples become stronger and more able to deepen their faith through their suffering. In Buddhism, suffering is necessary and requisite to being human, and is a part of the cycle of life. Suffering, in many religious contexts, is to be borne and by bearing it, it can be transcended (Halifax, 2009).

Bereavement scholars have written extensively about the suffering involved in grief. Many scholars note that suffering can be transformative, changing the mourner in positive ways (Neimeyer, 2001; Tedeschi and Calhoun, 2004). Freud (1917), in *Mourning and Melancholia*, and later in *The Ego and The Id* (1923), wrote that the ego of the bereaved person is always transformed by the nature of any loss, for better or for worse. Who we are is changed by the quality of the real relationships we have had with those we lose. Those real relationships become internalized and live on inside us as ghosts and ancestors after a person dies. In mourning, Freud wrote, a person's world is empty. In melancholia it is the self, or ego, that is empty and depleted. When we lose someone, whether the relationship was positive or negative, we internalize parts of the lost object. The ego of the survivor is forever changed as a result. Loewald (1962) noted that grief changes not only the mourner's ego, but also the mourner's superego. In our grief, he thought, we not only take in aspects of the person we have lost, but we also identify with the lost object's conscience and ideals. This leads to our own changed ideals, values and commitments based on the achievements of others. Out of suffering from grief, then, new purpose and meaning can develop (Berzoff, 2011). Neimeyer (2004) has further suggested that grief may be the occasion for post-traumatic growth. Tedeschi and Calhoun (2004) concur that the suffering in bereavement offers opportunities to shift priorities, make new meaning, and appreciate the preciousness of life. Growth – both psychic and emotional – might be called "learning from experience," the title of a book of essays by Bion (1984). Learning from experience is also a part of the endless repetitions of pain and suffering that both of my clients feel.

Egnew (2009) has written that suffering may simply need to be accepted, rather than transcended. Existentialists have contributed much to the knowledge of suffering. Victor Frankl, who survived the Holocaust in Auschwitz, wrote this,

> We must never forget that we may also find meaning in life even when confronted with a hopeless situation, when facing a fate that cannot be changed. For what then matters is to bear witness to the uniquely human potential at its best, which is to transform a personal tragedy into triumph, to turn one's predicament into a human achievement. When we are no longer able to change a situation – just think of an

> incurable disease such as inoperable cancer – we are challenged to change ourselves … When meaning can be assigned, the sufferer may even triumph.
>
> (1946, p. 135)

The question then arises about whether suffering must produce transformation or meaning (Rattner and Berzoff, 2016), or whether transformation and meaning idealize suffering? Writing about suffering at the end of life, Rattner and Berzoff (2018) question whether suffering is ennobling – or can even ever be fully integrated. In their counter-narrative, they ask about many forms of suffering in which no meaning can be found, no dignity gained. A child with an incurable disease, a needed young father with terminal testicular cancer, a teen killed in a bike accident, a heroin overdose by a promising young adult may intrinsically have no meaning.

> The wish to valorize all suffering as having the potential to change us may occur because it is so hard to sit with meaninglessness itself. It is difficult for patients, and their practitioners to deal with the fact that some suffering must simply be borne, by the patient, family and clinician.
>
> (Rattner and Berzoff, 2018)

Meaninglessness in relational work can be hard to bear.

Many authors have suggested that sitting with suffering requires sitting with our own mortality and with finitude. Currow and Hegarty (2006) write: "At very deep levels, real connection with a suffering person evokes in us the fear of our own undoing. It challenges us with the intimations of our own vulnerability and mortality" (as quoted in Rattner and Berzoff, 2016, p. 248).

Anatole Broyard, a literary critic diagnosed with metastatic prostate cancer, described facing his own mortality in his compelling memoir, *Intoxicated by My Illness* (1992). As he sought to find a relationship with a compassionate doctor who could bear his suffering, he wrote that he wanted to find someone who fully engaged him. He thought that all cures were actually talking cures. "The doctor has little to lose and much to gain by letting the sick man into his heart. If he does, they can share wonder, terror and the exaltation of being on the edge of being …" (Broyard, 1992, p. 57).

What Broyard also wanted was a practitioner who could simply allow him into his heart. This would require the doctor/helper to face her own mortality and deal with her own undoing. For practitioners, this is scary stuff. Do we, as practitioners, want to venture to the edge of being? Do we want to grapple with our own mortality and beyond?

Sitting with suffering, then, elicits helplessness and even despair in the clinician. Sitting with my client whose history of racism and child abuse makes him feel utterly unworthy of love induces helplessness in me. Sitting with my client who faces deportation, the loss of her child, and the loss of the productive and meaningful life she has constructed in this country, makes me feel impotent. My two early morning clients' losses and traumas: beatings, kidnappings, sexual abuse, the capriciousness of authoritarian regimes and families, exhaust me, empty me out. I feel great sorrow in the face of so much sorrow. A part of my sorrow is a projective identification. That is to say, how both clients unconsciously convey their pain is by inducing it in me. In our relational experience, I experience what cannot be said, but can be felt. How does any therapist hold so much pain and helplessness?

Back, Rushton, Kaszniak, and Halifax (2015) suggest that these moments of helplessness are precisely the moments of relationality. They reframe helplessness from

> being a soft underbelly that must be hidden, to an essential connection with the tragedy and fragility of being human. With clients who suffer, we are inevitably brought back to experiencing our own fragility and our own finitude. We are brought to into those feelings from our own tragedies, as part of the human condition.
>
> (2015, p. 27)

How do we stay with our clients' suffering? Many who write about suffering (Broyard, 1992; de Zulueta, 2015; Halifax, 2009) speak to imagination as the key. We need to be able to imagine our way into suffering because we cannot, as practitioners, have suffered in all the ways that our clients have. Broyard adds that imagination is a form of empathy. "Empathy is the imaginative identification with something we intuit in another person's psychological experience. This identification then becomes real to us" (as quoted by Harris, 2003, p. 101). Hannah Arendt wrote that Eichmann could perpetuate mass suffering precisely because he could not empathize or put himself in the shoes of another (2006). Levinas (1988), mentioned earlier, demands that empathy to suffering is our responsibility and duty.

DasGupta (2008), a palliative care physician, adds another component. While cultures, languages, races, genders may differ between client and clinician, the clinician must not only see but be seen, and by doing so enable herself to be seen more clearly. In sitting with suffering there are two interacting subjectivities, then, between client and clinician. Each must be able to feel what the other experiences and both must be receptive to one another. How do we let ourselves be seen?

My South African client often says to me, "You cannot know how I have suffered. You cannot possibly know what it is to be beaten or burned or hungry. You cannot know what it is to be unloved."

What is my response? Is it to tell him that I have suffered too? Is it to trot out my own losses, hurts, threats to my own integrity, so that he feels joined and understood? I think not. Instead, I feel with him his sorrow, his anger and grief. In Latin, "*compassion*" means "co-feeling." *Compassion* involves "feeling for another." His suffering needs to be felt, accepted, though not necessarily transcended or transformed (Egnew, 2009; Rattner and Berzoff, 2016). As his therapist, I need to be willing to share his pain and vulnerability. I need to go where it is uncomfortable, even unbearable – and find ways to bear it. Blum wrote

> Compassion is not simply a feeling state but a complex emotional attitude toward another, characteristically involving imaginative dwelling on the condition of the other person, an active regard for his good, a view of him as a fellow human being, and emotional responses of a certain degree of intensity.
>
> (Blum, 1980, p. 509)

We cannot sit with suffering in the cool space of neutrality. I have to feel my client's brokenness and my own. In fact, Rezenbrink (2017) says that "Compassion asks us to go where it hurts, to enter into places of pain, to share in brokenness, fear, confusion and anguish" (p. 247). A compassionate response is an active one. She quotes Nouwen and writes, "To the suffering of our clients, then, we bring our own active minds and experience," (p. 248).

When my client speaks of not having seen her father in 20 years, I feel the loss filtered through the loss of my own father in adolescence. When she talks about the disappearance of her sister when she was a young adolescent, I carry a lost sister in me. I don't need to talk about these losses. But they are there, parts of myself accessible to me as I sit with her. When my South African client cries quietly, "I am nothing. I am nobody," I feel those parts of myself in those times when I too have been brought to my knees with brokenness.

But I have had other resources to draw upon in my life that these clients have not. Robert Stolorow in an interview with Baer (2017) says this,

> Sharing the pain and providing a place where it can be helps to make it more bearable. It doesn't lessen the pain. In fact, in a way it could increase the pain, because it has a place where it's allowed to be, and where it could be shared. So it becomes more bearable.
>
> (p. 1)

There is something about sharing the pain in a therapeutic encounter, however intense it might be, which helps it become bearable precisely because the therapist is not overwhelmed or defensively shut down in the face of it.

David Browning (2004) reminds us that in our work with those who are suffering all we really have to bring is our own openness and moments of brokenness. Writing about a bereaved young girl whose sister had died, he remembers hoping to see her longer than the 12 sessions when she announced that she was ready to terminate. She reassured him, when he felt that they needed to work longer, that she was ready to end. She said that she carried two buckets of tears: a little bucket and a big bucket. While parents, teachers, friends and her therapist had helped her to empty the little bucket, she knew that she would always carry the big bucket of suffering alone. Browning goes on to say,

> In the most basic human sense, when we sit with another who is suffering, the only thing we truly have to offer is our own knowledge of suffering, our own wounds, our own broken hearts. Paradoxically, as we recognize our mutual vulnerability, we may help our clients find the strength to carry their buckets as they help us to find the strength to carry our own.
> (2004, p. 40)

This is a wonderfully realistic acknowledgement that in our work with clients, mourning may occur; suffering may be shared, grief may even be alleviated, but still clients will always carry their own grief and suffering, making suffering, in some ways, interminable.

Sitting with suffering in long-term relational practice

How do we sit with interminable suffering without burning out? How do we listen to the pain of our clients: racial, cultural, interpersonal and intrapsychic without becoming traumatized ourselves? There is a vast literature on compassion fatigue that I have previously reviewed (Berzoff and Kita, 2010). Halifax (2018) writes of compassion fatigue as altruism overload. According to Figley (2002), *compassion fatigue* is the reaction that emerges from the therapist's overexposure to client suffering: human brutality, war, disasters, loss, illness, rape, and other catastrophes. The clinician's overexposure is cumulative and takes place over extended periods of time (Adams, Boscarino, and Figley, 2006; Figley, 2002). Obviously the traumatic experiences of our clients weigh on us in ways that can undermine our own professional identities and personal lives. We may become depressed, we may burn out, we may forget things, we may want to turn away, we may even blame the victim. We may become angry, eat too much, eat too little, drink too much. Compassion may be hard to find, and we may want to tune out stories of hurt and pain. We may withdraw or find reasons to terminate early.

How do we maintain compassion and sit with suffering without compassion fatigue? First, we must be very well trained. By this I mean that we must know ourselves and our suffering well, and have the resilience to bear our own so that we do not burden our clients. Second, we need to have supervision and/or therapy that helps us to know and to hold our own suffering. Third, we need to be able to share the suffering with valued colleagues. In supervision groups that are peer-led, our authentic responses can emerge and we can collaborate about suffering. We can bring our countertransference responses to the group. For example, I talk about the pain I feel sitting with my South African client and, in sharing it, and in having my colleagues hold it, I can think about it. I can name it and experience it in more manageable forms. Writing in journals or writing for publication offers ways to share suffering. Likewise teaching can allow a practitioner to articulate her suffering in the face of her clients', in the presence of others, and thus feel less alone. Rezenbrink again, writes:

> The extent to which compassionate involvement can be sustained will depend on many things, including the resources available to us in the workplace as we struggle to make sense of tragedy. Skilled supervision and support from our superiors and colleagues can help us to set realistic goals and acknowledge our achievements. We will need a balanced workload with opportunities for creativity or "something for the soul" as a wise senior social worker once suggested. Sometimes there will be a need for personal therapy and healing activities such as meditation or other spiritual practices. At other times, "time out", physical exercise and laughter with family and friends will alleviate stress and cast away thoughts of difficult work encounters. Most importantly and often neglected is the grieving that we need to do ourselves, not only for the actual or fantasized deaths of people close to us but also for the little deaths or dyings we experience in life. The poet Kenneth Patchen (1936, p. 3) captures this idea perfectly with the words "There are so many little dyings, it doesn't matter which one of them is death".
>
> (2017, p. 247)

So how do I, on a Monday morning, find the fortitude to bear the suffering of two clients, back to back? First, I try to be present. Second, I bring some of my own loss and anguish from my own past (along with the repairs I have made along the way) to the experience. I try to listen with the sense that I have been there too. I also try to bring my strength, my knowledge, my training, my therapy, and experience to make the suffering thinkable. I have to be able, based on my training and experience, to maintain my own self and my own mind. If I lose my boundaries, as a clinician, I am not of use to my clients.

I also mix it up. If I see two people who are suffering profoundly, I will schedule two other patients with whom I can laugh because there is something quite wonderful about being able to laugh out loud at some of life's indignities. I will be sure to take a walk. I will have lunch with a friend. I will read a novel for a bit between clients. I will talk to colleagues. I will attend a group. I will write. I will teach. I will try to get outside of myself, gain perspective, touch base with those I love including my own children. In short, I will invest in the living to give me the fortitude and the strength to reconnect with the deepest parts of my own finitude.

Conclusion

In long-term relational practice with those who suffer, the practitioner is always changed by the work. When we sit with suffering we are brought into direct contact with human cruelty, loss, brutality and mortality. We are forced to reckon with the chaos that is out there. As we connect to the other, we experience not only our brokenness but also our survival, and not only the losses that have accrued to our clients but also their strengths. When our clients suffer, we also suffer. When they survive, we survive. When we survive, they can also. There is resilience that may emerge in a bidirectional relationship in which pain is borne with another. There is strength that comes with surviving suffering without cutting off the other as my South African client has had to do in the past.

My South African client comes in again. He tells me of an incident with one of his daughters who has refused to see him, text or take his calls. She is angry that he continues to want a relationship with her. I listen as he describes the loss of his three children. I imagine the loss as my own. It is incalculably difficult, but I see also see a tiny flicker of pleasure as he tells me of a success professionally. I think, "He is alive; he has survived, we will survive." My Palestinian client returns. Her daughter will stay in the US, and she will attend college while living with one of her friends. My client will return to Palestine. Again, I try to imagine what it is like to be forced to leave one's country, to leave one's child. I don't have to say that I am imagining her suffering. In the moment both of us are in it. But I also know that this client has faced the odds before and I know what strength lies within her. I believe that she does too. Over the years, her suffering has become more manageable. Together, in our experiencing it, her suffering is thinkable and, in that way, at times, almost bearable.

Sitting with another who suffers may offer both the practitioner and client hope that what exists can be borne. Perhaps what draws us to this work in the first place is that it connects us to what is possible. When we sit with suffering, we are confronted by that which we most fear and yet paradoxically, we may, by being present, become slightly more comfortable with the very worst that can happen. If our clients survive, so might we.

Henri Nouwen (1992), a theologist who wrote about suffering for practitioners said this:

> My own experience with anguish has been that facing it and living it through is the way to healing. But I cannot do that on my own. I need someone to keep me standing in it, to assure me that there is peace beyond the anguish, life beyond the death, and love beyond the fear. But I know now, at least, that attempting to avoid, repress, or escape the pain is like cutting off a limb that could be healed with proper attention. The deep truth is that our human suffering need not be an

> obstacle to the joy and peace we so desire, but can become, instead, the means to it … Real care means the willingness to help each other in making our brokenness into the gateway to joy.
>
> (p. 87)

I am going on a five-week vacation and to a writing retreat in Italy. My South African client comes to the third to the last session before I leave. He hands me a book on the Holocaust and asks me to read it. I am preoccupied with leaving, with packing and with the details of travel. I have recently foresworn any more Holocaust books. They are simply too unbearable to hold these days. I say that I will try to get to it. In fact, I don't. It is not until I return five weeks later that I finally read the book. It ends, in a paraphrased way, with a paragraph that says that despite the Nazis finding ways to kill and destroy us, despite their trying to wipe us off of the face of the earth, we are still here; we are still here. I am stunned that this is the message of the book, that hope exists, and that suffering can be borne. This conviction, expressed between us at different moments in the treatment, I believe, is at the heart of long-term relational practice and is what, in the end, may help us all survive.

References

Adams, R., Boscarino, J. A. and Figley, C. (2006). Compassion fatigue and psychological distress among social workers: A validation study. *American Journal of Orthopsychiatry*, 76, 103–108.

Arendt, H. (2006). *Eichmann on Jerusalem: A report on the banality of evil*. New York, NY: Penguin.

Back, A. L., Rushton, C. H., Kaszniak, A. W. and Halifax, J. S. (2015). "Why are we doing this?" Clinician helplessness in the face of suffering. *Journal of Palliative Medicine*, 18 (1), 26–30.

Baer, D. (2017, September 26). Why you should never tell someone who's grieving to "move on": Instead of pushing their pain away, lean into it. *Thrive Global*. Thriveglobal.com/stories/14014.

Berzoff, J. (2011). The transformative nature of grief and bereavement. *Clinical Social Work Journal*, 39 (3), 262–269.

Berzoff, J. and Kita, E. (2010). Compassion fatigue and countertransference: Two different concepts. *Clinical Social Work Journal*, 38 (3), 341–349.

Bion, W. R. (1984). *Learning from experience*. London: Karnac.

Blum, L. (1980). Compassion. In A. O. Rorty (Ed.), *Explaining emotions*. Berkeley, CA: University of California Press, 507–519.

Browning, D. (2004). Fragments of love: Explorations in the ethnography of suffering and professional caregiving. In J. Berzoff and P. Silverman (Eds.), *Living with dying: A handbook for end-of-life healthcare practitioners*. New York, NY: Columbia University Press, 21–42.

Broyard, A. (1992). *Intoxicated by my illness: And other writings on life and death*. New York, NY: Clarkson Potter.

Currow, D. C. and Hegarty, M. (2006). Residential aged-care facility palliative care guidelines: Improving care. *International Journal of Palliative Care*, 12 (5), 231–233.
DasGupta, S. (2008). Narrative humility. *The Lancet*, 371 (9617), 980–981.
Davies, J. (2011). Positive and negative models of suffering: An anthropology of our shifting cultural consciousness of emotional discontent. *Anthropology of Consciousness*, 22 (2), 188–208.
de Zulueta, P. C. (2015). Suffering, compassion and "doing good medical ethics" *Journal of Medical Ethics*, 41, 87–90.
Egnew, T. R. (2009). Suffering, meaning, and healing: Challenges of contemporary medicine. *Annals of Family Medicine*, 7 (2), 170–175.
Figley, C. R. (2002). Compassion fatigue: Psychotherapists' chronic lack of self care. *Journal of Clinical Psychology*, 58 (11), 1433–1441.
Frank, A. W. (1995). *The wounded storyteller: Body, illness, and ethics*. Chicago, IL: University of Chicago Press.
Frankl, V. (1946). *Man's search for meaning*. Boston, MA: Beacon Press.
Freud, S. (1917). Mourning and melancholia. In *The standard edition of the complete psychological works of Sigmund Freud*, vol. 14. London: Hogarth Press, 237–258.
Freud, S. (1923). *The ego and the id*. London: Hogarth Press.
Green, R. and Palpant, N. (Eds.). (2014). *Suffering and bioethics*. New York, NY: Oxford University Press.
Halifax, J. (2009). *Being with dying: Cultivating compassion and fearlessness in the presence of death*. Boston, MA: Shambala.
Halifax, J. (2018). *Standing at the edge: Finding freedom where fear and courage meet*. New York, NY: Macmillan
Harris, J. (2003). *Signifying pain: Constructing and healing the self through writing*. Albany, NY: State University of New York Press.
Levinas, E. (1988). Useless suffering. In R. Bernasconi and D. Wood (Eds.), *The provocation of Levinas: Rethinking the other*. New York, NY: Routledge, 156–166.
Loewald, H. (1962). Internalization, separation and mourning and the superego. *Psychoanalytic Quarterly*, 31, 453–504.
Neimeyer, R. A. (2001). *Meaning reconstruction and the experience of loss*. Washington, DC: American Psychological Association.
Neimeyer, R. A. (2004). Fostering posttraumatic growth: A narrative elaboration. *Psychological Inquiry*, 15 (1), 53–59.
Nouwen, H. (1979). *The wounded healer: Ministry in contemporary society*. New York, NY: Random House.
Nouwen, H. (1992). *Life of the beloved: Spiritual living in a secular world*. New York, NY: Crossroads.
Patchen, K. (1936). *Selected poems by Kenneth Patchen*. New York, NY: Modern Library.
Rattner, M. and Berzoff, J. (2016). Rethinking suffering: Allowing for suffering that is intrinsic at the end of life. *Journal of Social Work in End-of-Life & Palliative Care*, 12 (3), 240–258.
Rattner, M. and Berzoff, J. (2018). Sitting with suffering in end of life care. *Journal of Palliative Care*, under review.

Rezenbrink, I. (2017). Suffering in end of life care: An arts-based approach. In B. Crisp (Ed.), *The routledge handbook of religion, spirituality and social work*. New York, NY: Routledge, 245–253.

Tedeschi, R. G. and Calhoun, L. G. (2004). Posttraumatic growth: Conceptual foundations and empirical evidence. *Psychological Inquiry*, 15 (1), 1–18.

Wilt, J. A., Exline, J. J., Lindberg, M. J., Park, C. L. and Pargament, K. I. (2017). Theological beliefs about suffering and interactions with the divine. *Psychology of Religion and Spirituality*, 9, 137–147. doi:10.1037/rel0000067.

Chapter 11

Till death do us part

Relational work and terminal illness

Susan Lord

I had forgotten what it felt like to sit with her. That feeling of darkness, of isolation, her rage seething just below the surface. I could feel myself shrinking, trying to become smaller so as not to interfere with her process as she sat there with her g-tube and pump, the bag of dark outflow hanging from the back of her chair.

She was 63, the age that my analyst had been when he died of the same illness long before we were done with our work. The age that her father had been when he died of a heart attack when she was in her twenties. My age. She and I had been working together two or three times each week for 24 years, and had terminated successfully/joyfully only nine months ago. I received a message from her in August saying that she would like to talk with me about "some changes that are happening in my life".

Stage four cancer. She could not come to me as she was in too much pain and the long drive was more than she could handle even with someone driving her, and so I offered to come to her. We met in her home office. I was anxious, distracted by seeing her in her home, a place that I had been hearing about for years. It was smaller, darker than I had imagined. I was worried about boundaries and about the volatility of my emotions. This was so sad. So unfair. So final. I felt helpless, guilty about my good health and larger-than-life robust energy.

And so we began again, although the territory was very different. We were headed not toward a future, but toward her end. She met me at the door with no greeting; there was no feeling of connection, though we hadn't seen each other for nine months. She motioned for me to follow her down a flight of stairs into her cold dark office. She walked slowly and painfully to her seat where she carefully laid out her paraphernalia. She had learned of her terminal diagnosis two weeks before, and had just been discharged from the hospital where she had undergone an emergency surgery.

In a hoarse voice she told me that she was struggling with feeling that she had failed. She had "not been in touch with her body" and, had she "taken herself more seriously", she would have sought medical treatment sooner. When she did go, her doctor had also not taken her symptoms seriously and had told her to exercise more and to be more careful with her diet. She said that she was feeling shame and guilt, as she had always wanted to die and had wished for a cancer diagnosis so that she wouldn't have to be responsible for her death. "In many ways", she said, "I feel relieved and I want this to be over with as quickly as possible". "I've had a good life, though it has been a struggle". This, she said, was why she had decided to contact me again. I was the only person that she could talk with about these things.

As we settled into the session and our new "normal", my phone made a sound as I received a text. That I had not turned off my phone was another sign that I was rattled. I apologized, and she looked down and pulled inward as if to gather herself. I could feel her anger coming at me from across the room; a palpable wave of energy pushing me backward in my chair. I had forgotten what it felt like to sit with her. And this was different. She felt more measured, more controlled, more rageful, more controlling of me.

This is a chapter about a long-term relational psychotherapy that will likely end with the death of my client before this book is published. I would like to write about our process as we move through this most human of journeys together.

Background

The psychotherapeutic relationship is one that, by its very definition, is the most real and the most unreal relationship that any of us may have the privilege to participate in. It is out of time and space, protected by the parameters of a frame, and limited and limitless in its capacities to engender trust, holding, and intensified processes of growth and change.

Bergmann spoke of the significance of the therapeutic relationship, and the ironic abruptness with which therapies end:

> In real life we encounter three types of termination of human relationships; geographical separation, transformation of a friendly or love relationship into a hostile one, and death. The analysand, however, is supposed to bring about separation under conditions of love and gratitude … Under these conditions, an analysis is exceptionally difficult to end, for patient and analyst alike.
>
> (1997, p. 168)

Long-term work that ends with the death of one's client offers a particularly poignant crucible upon which to develop and process mutual intimacies. Byock (1997) has written,

> Being present when someone is dying tears the boundaries between the personal and the professional realms of my being. The experience of

> a patient dying challenges me to accept a more intimate, and yet more deeply respectful, relationship with that person. I do not know how it could be otherwise. While I may bring clinical skills and years of experience to the task, ultimately I am simply present, offering to help and wanting to learn.
>
> (p. XIV)

L.

Upon receiving the call from L., I found that I was extremely anxious about the decision to continue our work together. I had, throughout our 24 years together, had a love/hate relationship with her, and our ending had felt powerful, positive, and final. I consulted with colleagues as I prepared to venture into this unknown territory.

I combed the literature, reviewing such touchstones as Kubler-Ross's *On Death and Dying* (1969) and *Living with Death and Dying* (1981), Berzoff and Silverman's very helpful *Handbook for End-of-Life Practitioners* (2004), Mayer's "Implications for Psychoanalytic Technique Drawn from Analysis of a Dying Patient" (1994), Edwards's "The Ailing Analyst and the Dying Patient" (2004) and Redding's "When Death Becomes the End of an Analytic Treatment" (2005). Their wisdom shored me up with the consistent message that there was no "right" way to do this work, and that going with the flow in a way that was ethical, mutually respectful and accommodating of the inevitable changes as they happened was what was indicated. What seemed most important were presence, empathy and compassion, and flexibility as I entered into this new relationship.

A change in frame

Somehow the frame has changed and structures need to be flexible, accommodating the ebbs and flows of energy, L's medical situation (chemotherapy schedule, hospitalizations), and psychic availability. While in many ways she is more available for intimate discourse, she is sometimes just unable to participate. We settle into a schedule in which she calls the shots. Slavin has written about the need to alter the frame "toward a form that is much more closely aligned with the realities of a particular patient's life, needs, and interests" (2001, p. 421). We commit to meeting every two-to-three weeks if possible, and meeting more or less frequently as needed.

The arc of our work together

Throughout our 24 years of work together we have gone through many changes, both of us, weathered many storms, both of us, and grown and changed in many ways, together and apart.

L. began with me in a state of regression. She was referred by her couple therapist, as she had recovered memories of childhood sexual abuse while trying to work on her sexual relationship (or lack thereof) with her partner. For the first two years of our work together she would arrive at my office, curl up into a ball on the couch, and rock. In her life out there in the world she functioned very well. She was in a high-powered and responsible position at work, and there was never a problem there. Somehow she was able to pull herself together and perform beautifully at a job that required much of her. It was difficult for me to believe that she could do so well, when she was struggling to even communicate with me in the office.

In a sense, we had grown up together. Several years into our work I moved my office to another city an hour away. She followed me there, committing to drive a two-hour round-trip twice a week. She had moved along in her life to a point at which she had developed internal structure and flexibility. She had mourned the loss of her father, and had come to terms with her intrusive, controlling and abusive mother. Although her difficulties with her sexual self had kept her in treatment for all of those many years, she had made tremendous gains in every other area of her life. She no longer had suicidal thoughts, she had stopped her self-harming behaviors, had come to terms with her difficulties with emotional intimacy and was at peace with her life. And so we terminated.

And now, as we begin again, I am driving to her, and meeting with her in her space. I am amazed that she was able to devote three hours two times each week to our work for so many years.

Repulsion and anxiety

As I drive toward her, I am filled with anxiety and repulsion. Will I be able to stomach all of this? The smells, the sounds. The visuals as she fades away, her features becoming sunken, her body wasting. I have worked with people with AIDS, and have done some hospice work in the past, but this is different. L. is a person with whom I have had a relationship, albeit a therapeutic one, for 24 years.

When my mother died, when my sister died, I could handle everything and anything because of my love for them. I didn't see things. Right up until the last day, for each of them, I was oblivious to the physical details of their dying processes. I saw only them, shining through. I did, on the last day, feel repulsed. I can vividly remember rushing home to wash the feelings, smells, and visual images of death away in a long hot shower. This is where I began with L. My awareness of everything was heightened.

My analyst's death was one in which I didn't participate. I received the call from his wife saying that he would not be returning to his practice. Each week I dropped off containers of healing teas that I had made for him in attempts to ease his pain, cure the cancer; she graciously accepted them and said that he found them soothing. I wrote to him, telling him that I was okay, that we had done the work we needed to do and that I would have continued to see him forever because I found it helpful and loved him and felt loved by him. I told him that my only wish was that he not be afraid and not be in pain. I saw him once more several months before he died and we were able to say goodbye.

This death is most similar to his. L. has the same diagnosis. The same prognosis. This may be an opportunity for me to bear witness to that which I could not be part of before. A double-edged sword for me. I can already feel myself shrinking from the physical realities of her dying process in ways I never have before.

Bromberg has written about how important it is to accept the patient "on his own terms, and at the same time not settle for them" (1998, p. 20). During our entire relationship I have had a vision of L. and of her life as bigger than it actually is. This, in a way, has served to broaden our work together. Somehow the reality of the narrowness and darkness of her world has hit me hard. The planes of her lived experience are not as I had imagined them to be, and I feel our work diminished by the realities of this. I had projected light and air and space into her stuffy and narrow realities.

Diminishment

"Would you like me to turn on the air? It feels close in here. I get overheated easily now". L. sits across from me, diminished. She has lost all of her hair, and about 30 pounds. She was already thin, and her appearance is now one of a wizened older woman. She has gone through one round of chemotherapy and is trying to decide whether quality of life is more important than gaining more time. She won't know until after the second round whether the chemo is working, and so she has decided to go through with that at least.

Bearing witness

She uses our time together to talk about her ambivalence about living. She has, for as long as she can remember, experienced her life as something she must endure. She grew up in a family that she describes as harsh and narrow. Her parents were strictly religious Lutherans, and were exacting in their requirements and criticisms of her and her two siblings. She tried always to "be good" and to "do the right thing". She and her siblings have all lived limited small and joyless lives.

She has also spent her life negotiating the terrain of trauma. As the oldest, she was the target of her now-89-year-old mother's physical and sexual abuse when she was an infant. She has shadowed memories of pain, and clearer memories of an always-conflicted relationship with her mother. Her father was more loving and available, though he died when she was in her twenties. In our work together she has been able to negotiate a closer relationship with her mother, though she remains hypervigilant and prepared for inevitable strife.

She is planning to invite her family to her home for a final Christmas together, and is hoping that her mother will be able to make the long trip. "How strange that I will be dying before my mother does."

Grief and loss: embracing despair

She tells me that she is upset about all of the people who are "coming out of the woodwork" to see her. Many of them she has not seen in years. It is hard to see them go through their grief processes, as she is beyond where they are and has accepted that she is going to die. She finds herself wishing that they would leave, and wondering about the sincerity of their grief. "It all seems to be about them, not about me and my process." I am reminded of vultures circling.

Confessor

I find myself feeling that I am her confessor. I will go to the grave holding her secrets. L. says that she needs to continue working with me as I am the only person that she is able to talk with about certain things. She says that she has always wanted to die. That she is glad that she will never have to have sex again. She misses the pleasure of eating, but many of the trappings of her life have been difficult for her.

Midwife

I have an awareness of the similarities between the beginnings and endings of our lives. We gather as families and communities to welcome a newcomer into the world, just as we gather to bear witness to the end of a life. It seems that we generally die as we have lived. There are opportunities here, to say what needs to be said and do what needs to be done. And there are enormous opportunities to change things.

My job, it seems, has changed to that of midwife. We are no longer client and psychotherapist. We are two human beings in a room. Hearts beating, energies in sync. I am aware of the gifts of this process; the moment-to-moment heightened awareness of what matters. What matters is what matters at the moment; all else falls away. In so many ways death teaches us how to live. Sparely, to the bone.

For L., for whom any form of intimacy has been fraught with dangerous traps, this business of dying is more than difficult. She has become a "sitting duck" – a "target" for those who want to visit and help and offer their love.

She and I need to be careful to not fall into patterns in which she accommodates me and takes care of my needs. L. has said that she is not a spiritual person; she believes in nothing. Nature, however, has always called to her and she has been able to find a semblance of peace and comfort there. Music has also been very important in her life. Her mother was a music teacher, and so music is mixed for her. She has had some self-punitive ideas about perfection and discipline when she makes music. She plays the cello, and is in a professional orchestra. She has had to give up the orchestra as she has become more ill. Music does still have the ability to transport her to different states of being. I encourage her to remember to listen to music as much as possible, and to look out the window at the birds, at nature.

Falling away

"I feel myself becoming detached from most things, and from people. Yet it is hard to let go of things." L. talks about the fact that most of her clothes no longer fit. She is reluctant to give away her clothes – to acknowledge that she will never regain the weight she has lost. She is also reluctant to buy new clothes as she has no plans to go anywhere.

She is clear that there are places that she will never visit, dreams she will never fulfill. She becomes tearful as she talks about never seeing the Pacific Ocean again. She will never again walk on the beach near my office, as she used to before our sessions.

Her mother has decided that she cannot travel to visit L., and so she has seen her mother for the last time. They talk regularly on the phone, but have "nothing to say to each other", as their lives have become ironically similar. Neither goes anywhere or does anything. Both are in pain and are witnessing their worlds growing smaller.

She feels her interests falling away, and wonders whether she is depressed. Is it her illness? I suggest that it might be that she is disengaging from the world. There is a kind of anesthesia that begins to happen as people are preparing for death. She says that she feels it is more about focusing on presence and on truths, on what is important. She has no time to waste and she is clearer and beginning to live more authentically, from the inside out.

What is important

L. is beginning to separate out what is important to her and what is not. Ironically, as her life is coming to a close, she is finding that she feels more alive. She is able to feel loved and to engage more fully with people. She says that she doesn't feel that constant anxiety about all that she needs to do, and is beginning to be able to "just be". I notice that her restlessness and subtle self-harming behaviors have all but disappeared. She used to subtly scratch her legs or pinch the palms of her hands as she sat with me; her legs were restless and she would fidget and have a hard time sitting still. She used to tell me about "night terrors" in which she would cry out in her sleep and awaken in a panic that she had forgotten to feed some tiny animal and it would die. She seems now to be inhabiting her Self, and her life in a different way.

Moments of meeting

I am finding that it is becoming more difficult for me to end each session. In my office, beginnings and endings have always been on the dot, a practice that clients have said they found both rigid and comforting, organizing, creating a sense of safety and firm boundaries. As I gather myself to leave, I find that I am more and more reluctant to end things. I stand at the doorway and say, "you are handling all of this with such grace and courage". Her eyes tear up, as do mine.

She has only cried with me two or three times in all of the years, and this feels like such a gift as I find my way out and walk to my car.

I am dying

L says, "I walk around and every so often the thought pops into my head: 'I am dying'. I think about whether it will hurt. How will it happen? I feel like I am wasting time".

It is March and she learns that the chemotherapy is no longer working and posts a note on her CaringBridge site,

> Well, the news is not good. The reason that my liver enzymes are up is because the metastases in my liver are getting bigger and more numerous, and are causing some blockage of the bile ducts in the liver. There are also clearly metastases in my lungs ... All of this is very scary and upsetting ... I can't emphasize enough how much all of you have given us through your loving comments, emails, flowers, gifts, cards, visits, transportation, and phone calls. Thank you from my over-flowing heart.

Her raw honesty, vulnerability and expansiveness are palpable. I now find myself looking forward to our sessions. I am no longer repulsed, and it seems I will be able to handle everything and anything that might come. As with other loved ones who have died, I no longer see things. I have become oblivious to the physical details of her dying process. L. is more available and there is a sweetness to the sorrow of what is happening. I am told by a colleague that I must prepare myself for the possibility that she will need to pull away from me before she dies. The oncologist has given her a range of time to anticipate, maybe six months at the outside. We are now seven months in from diagnosis, and she believes she was symptomatic for several months before that. We are running out of time.

Addendum: L. died in July, almost a year after she was diagnosed with pancreatic cancer. We had our last session just hours before she died and were able to say goodbye.

References

Bergmann, M. S. (1997). Termination: The Achilles heel of psychoanalytic technique. *Psychoanalytic Psychology, 14*, 163–174.

Berzoff, J. & Silverman, P. R. (2004). *Living with dying: A handbook for end-of-life healthcare practitioners.* New York, NY: Columbia University Press.

Bromberg, P. M. (1998). *Standing in the spaces: Essays on clinical process, trauma, and dissociation.* Hillsdale, NJ: The Analytic Press.

Byock, I. (1997). *Dying well: Peace and possibilities at the end of life.* New York, NY: Riverhead Books.

Edwards, N. (2004). The ailing analyst and the dying patient: A relational perspective. *Psychoanalytic Dialogues, 14*(3), 313–335.

Kubler-Ross, E. (1969). *On death and dying.* New York, NY: Simon & Schuster.

Kubler-Ross, E. (1981). *Living with death and dying.* New York, NY: Macmillan.

Mayer, E. (1994). Some implications for psychoanalytic technique drawn from analysis of a dying patient. *Psychoanalytic Quarterly, 63*, 1–19.

Redding, K. K. (2005). When death becomes the end of an analytic treatment: Necessary parameters. *Clinical Social Work Journal, 33*(1), 69–79.

Slavin, M. (2001). Review essay: Constructivism with a human face. *Psychoanalytic Dialogues, 11*, 405–429.

Chapter 12

Looking back through 38 years of practicing relational psychoanalysis in search of answers to the question of interminability

Stefanie Solow Glennon

Earlier this year I received an e-mail from Dr. Susan Lord letting me know that she was editing a forthcoming book with the working title *Relational Therapy Interminable?* She was interested in the question I had posed previously in a chapter entitled "Relational analyses: Are they more difficult to terminate?," and asked if I would consider writing a chapter for her book expanding on the topic. I happily agreed to do so.

To quote from that first chapter:

> In our increasingly relational world of psychoanalysis, I find myself troubled regarding the degree to which the intimacy and power of the relationship between patient and analyst can elongate the length of the treatment or even make termination unthinkable. If a patient has done a substantial piece of analytic work and is quite ready for the termination phase but feels reluctant to leave the relationship with the analyst because the relationship feels so good, is so meaningful, is one of love and caring, and because he or she feels so close to the analyst, whom he or she now knows quite intimately (given the openness and lack of anonymity with which most of us carry on our analytic work), then we have a problem. I am suggesting that the dilemma of finding the line to walk such that the relationship can sustain optimal therapeutic action, but at the same time be a relationship that one can willingly leave, is a difficult task.
>
> (Glennon, 2010)

The above thoughts were stimulated by a particularly difficult session around the issue of termination. The patient at the time was a 67-year-old woman with whom I had been working mainly in a three-times-a-week relational analysis for 21 years. I had been feeling for some time that since she had made significant changes in most of the important areas of her life, termination should be considered. I had actually been expecting her to bring it up. She didn't, so I did. Here is her response:

> Why would I even consider that? I have had enough losses in my life. Why would I *choose* to say goodbye to you? Why would I *choose* to sever a relationship that is so dear to me, so special and like none I've ever had before? It feels so unnatural. In life outside this office the only time a relationship like this would end would be due to death … It seems crazy to me. I can afford to come here. I have the time and the money, and I can't even imagine not seeing you anymore.

The patient is not in the field, so it is unlikely that our paths would cross after termination. She was adamant in her refusal to consider ending and I stopped bringing it up. We proceeded to go on with our work for another four years. It was shortly after this interaction that I wrote my previous chapter.

But what she had said in 2009 made sense to me in terms of the intensity and mutuality of our long relationship and I wondered if this were not a factor operating in long-term relational analyses making them more difficult to terminate. My thought was that if this was occurring in my practice with this very long-term patient, might it not be a generalizable phenomenon?

I subsequently conducted a search of the analytic literature to see if others had raised the question. The only relevant thinking I could find came from Martin Bergmann (1997) who said, "In real life, only death and hostility bring a libidinal relationship to an end. The kind of termination psychoanalysis demands is without precedent" (p. 173). But Bergmann did not raise the question as to whether or not a more intense, more personal, more "relational" analytic relationship might heighten or exacerbate the pain of termination and thereby result in interminability.

With Dr. Lord's question in mind regarding the extent to which relational analyses may be interminable – not just more difficult to terminate – I decided to look back within my 38-year practice to ferret out long-term analyses that had ended in "natural" terminations from those that had not, and therefore might be considered "interminable."

Somewhat surprisingly and relievedly I found that the great majority of long and very long-term analyses had ended in what would be considered successful terminations. As part of the termination process, most of these patients verbalized the difficulty of saying goodbye, but they were able and wanted to do so. This finding was relieving to me since I have not given up my conviction that being able to terminate and go on in life, maintaining the gains made in analysis without the analysis or analyst, is a process that carries its own benefits. One woman who terminated after 25 years said in our last session, "I don't feel afraid to be." I ran into her once and we hugged, looked deeply into each other's eyes, saw the connection and the old feelings still alive, and we never spoke again. That was about eight years ago now.

The patient who evoked these questions in my original paper has "opted" not to leave entirely (she comes in once a month), and for her I don't think the adjective "interminable" fits her situation. I agree with her that she has made a choice that does not reflect an inability. I asked if she would like to comment on what led to this decision and how it has played out for her. After some thought, she let me know that she would like to contribute to the chapter and her comments appear at the end.

A question that has arisen for me in the process of thinking about and researching my practice for data, is how to define "interminable." When do we hypothesize that a 10-year treatment, for example, might become interminable or might end in another five, ten or 15 years? I found in my look-back two 25-year analyses and a 20-year analysis, all of which ended well – with others ending after ten, 12, 13, 17, 18, and 19 years. Perhaps the conclusion to be drawn is that we cannot know, cannot even hypothesize, the length of any particular treatment or what factors will contribute to an inability to terminate.

"Interminable" implies something within the patient that makes the prospect of leaving the analyst too dangerous, too life-robbing, and therefore frightening. Extreme dependence and an inability to grasp the gifts of autonomy have been the usual culprits mentioned in the literature. Those were clearly not the underlying factors in my patient's not wanting to leave me, not wanting to say goodbye to Stefanie Glennon. Why she ultimately (after four more years) made the choice she did, i.e. to come in once a month, for checking in, wanting to know how I am, could be a cover for some sort of "inability" but it does not feel like that to me – or her. (She is an independent woman leading a full, active life with many close friends.) As she said in her statement quoted above, she can afford to come, is willing to pay for the ability to see me and continue what she had termed during our work, "the friendship part" without having a friendship in the usual sense outside of the office. I have told her, and she agrees, that doing so can damage gains made during the analysis and also, if something happens in the future that results in a desire to return to treatment, the friendship could make that no longer possible or optimal.

At some point in this process I decided to focus on current patients in long-term analyses for whom termination is not on the horizon and has not yet been mentioned by them or thought of by me. I naively wanted to see whether or not I could isolate some variables (amidst all the uniqueness of each individual and therefore each dyad) to account for the possibility that their treatments may result in being interminable.

At first I thought about the issue of their highly, unusually disturbed mothers and absent fathers. Then I realized that one of these patients had a father who was not emotionally absent but rather preferred her to her envious, emotionally self-absorbed, uninvolved mother. Besides, as I thought further, there had been many patients who had terminated who had had difficult mothers, and difficult fathers, in all sorts of degrees and permutations. I, not quickly enough, came to the conclusion that searching for commonalities in the psychodynamics of patients in long-term analyses who have not (yet) brought up or perhaps even thought about termination, is fruitless. To quote Ed Levenson (1976):

> I would say that it makes no more sense to ask when or how to terminate than to ask when to die. It is a natural event in the course of therapy … Every conceivable permutation and combination of position about the meaning of termination is represented in the psychoanalytic literature and one can find scriptures to one's purpose without any great difficulty.
>
> (p. 341)

What became obvious (and should have been expected) is that each of these patients (with perhaps one exception) "know" (in the unthought known sense that Bollas (1989) talks about) that there is more life-enhancing work to be done and that is the reason why neither I nor they have as yet had termination thoughts. In my view, for at least three of the four patients, interminability is not the issue.

There is, however, one woman who has been coming for 20 years, once a week, who has welcomed having someone "to talk with" (she has no friends) and though highly intelligent, has greeted any forays into interpretive work "as interesting" and then moved on. I have grappled with my own feelings of impotence and perhaps incompetence, and at one point suggested that perhaps she should see someone else since it seemed to me we were not making progress with her isolation and another disturbing, idiosyncratic symptom (which I will not go into because of confidentiality concerns), but she refused. My surmise is that there is feared to be unprocessable pain that is being held at bay. Perhaps if we had been able to work more frequently, we might have been able to move forward. But she has found reasons why that could not happen, and I have stopped making the suggestion. I have given up trying to explore, interpret, promote understanding and am just there – as spontaneously as I am able. That's all she seems to respond to.

I do care about her – she's right about that, but I'm also aware of an iciness, a wall beyond which I cannot go. Nonetheless she trusts me, feels better after we've "talked" and that's not nothing. My ambition for her – given how gifted she is – has had to be shelved. She has been married for many years. The relationship is stable but dutiful, polite, filled with a lot of talk, but little spontaneity. They share intellectual interests, but emotions are not allowed. Total mutual dependence is the sustaining core of their relationship. They've had no children.

I've gone into so much detail about the above patient not because our work is indicative of other long-term treatments, but rather because it is one that might very well be "interminable" and therefore unusual in my years of practice. The hurdle for me with her was continuing to see her, being paid by her, when I've felt that gains were so minimal. And then I realized I should trust her judgment that what we have IS important to her – perhaps even crucial, and just let it be.

My answer to the question I raised in my initial paper is, yes, relational analyses are likely "more difficult" to terminate. It is more difficult to say goodbye to someone now known so well, and so cared about, way beyond the blank screened or anonymous analyst of old. But being more difficult to terminate has not, in my experience, led to interminability. In addition, that increased difficulty is far outweighed by the therapeutic action that may only come from a long analytic relationship.

In a paper presented at a conference in New York this year, Tony Bass stated,

> I too believe that no small part of an analysis is the creation of new "objects", not only through the identification and interpretation of the sources of such internalized processes, but through experience that the relationship generates and how it contrasts with prior experience. I think this is one of the insufficiently considered aspects of long analysis. We often speak of the importance of so-called termination experience in analysis, and I agree that there is much to be mined there in regard to separation, individuation and autonomy. But I also think that long, productive analyses enrich lives in no small part through the creation of new histories, new internal object processes that constitute, in effect, internalizations of the therapeutic relationship. A patient of mine, in her third decade of analysis recently said that as the sessions and years add up, her experience with me begins to take on the weight of the years of experience prior to our analysis.
>
> (Bass, 2018)

I could not agree more, and find this to be a creative new thought about how the duration of the new object experience, in actual time, can in some cases be crucial in counteracting the old solidly implanted bad object relationship. There is something obvious in this conclusion that has been overlooked – perhaps because of the analyst's shame about long ongoing analyses; what might be said about the incompetence or lack of integrity of the analyst.

I am grateful to Dr. Susan Lord for her request which has resulted in my thinking further about relational analyses and the issue of terminability. Looking back over my clinical practice (which I would not have done) I have discovered that analyses that might along the way have seemed interminable (over ten years or more) did in fact end well and that only a few treatments may go on until "death do us part."

The increased difficulty in terminating relational treatment is, as Tony Bass pointed out, superseded by the increased gains of many years of an intense, mutually knowing and loving, intimate, yet professional relationship. I now think that eight years ago I was too quick to worry about the generalizability of my patient's ardently expressed response to termination and her refusal to even think about it. Her feelings made so much sense, given the nature of our relationship, that I feared similar feelings in others might make leaving impossible for them. Thankfully that has not been the case. Interminability is clearly linked to other variables.

Another issue

There is another issue that arose during the preparation of this chapter that I would like to share with my readers. In thinking that I would like input from a few other people who had successfully terminated long-term analyses, I called another person, someone with whom I had worked for 19 years and had not seen for more than eight years. I reached her on the phone and asked if she would be willing to write about her experience of our termination. I told her that, if she decided to do so, what she wrote would appear in a chapter I was writing. I of course asked her to be sure it was something she felt comfortable doing and, if not, I would fully understand and that would be fine. She readily agreed, without giving it further thought. We had a long phone conversation during which she told me of the problems she was having with her now grown son (I remembered holding him as an infant when she had brought him in during one of our early sessions). During this conversation I became aware that although she was open in what she had to say, there was a pressured quality and lack of ease that was different from our way of relating when we were working together. She was interested in the idea, is a talented, professional writer, and said she would be happy to contribute to the chapter. I e-mailed her my original article so that she would have an idea of my thinking.

Well over a month went by and I did not hear from her. I then e-mailed her and got a response telling me how involved with her son's difficulties she had been, apologizing for not letting me know, and stating she cannot do this now. I wrote back saying I fully understood and hoped that things with her son would work out well. I even had made a referral for rehab for him in our phone conversation. I asked her to let me know how things worked out. I haven't heard from her since. It's been a few months and my feeling is I will not hear from her – and it is not a good feeling.

Shortly after calling the above patient and before the denouement of that interaction, I e-mailed another person who readily agreed to write the response (entitled "Second Patient" which appears at the end of this chapter). After a few weeks, she wrote the following:

> Dear Stefanie,
> This has been complicated. Absorbing, but not simple. I've chosen not to write about my ambivalent response to your request – which began with my almost forgetting about it, then later discovering that I had, in fact, trashed your paper. When you asked me if I were interested, I was pleased and intrigued, but also (as a dream made clear) I felt angry, invaded, trapped and competitive. I'm sure that's another paper waiting to be written, but I don't want to write it. And this is surely not the place for it. I thought about mentioning it in my response, but that would risk opening a can of psychoanalytic worms that every reader would want elaborated. I decided to stick with my conscious experience of doing well without our sessions.

And then she included in her e-mail the thoughtful, beautiful piece which appears at the end of this paper. On some level I was pleased not only that she was aware of her ambivalent reaction, but that she could let me know.

The combination of the one patient's changing her mind about my request (and the way in which she handled that) and the ambivalent experience of the patient who did decide to write, has resulted in my coming to the conclusion that I will never do this again. I will never initiate contact – for whatever reason – with a patient who has successfully terminated, especially if it is to ask them to do me a favor. I had actually had in mind to contact another patient who had successfully terminated after 20 years, another articulate gifted writer, but after these two experiences I could not imagine risking "intruding" into her life, and didn't.

I have in the past had the thought of wanting to contact a patient just to find out how they are, missing them and wanting to catch up some, but I have resisted doing so for fear that it would open a door that had been carefully closed and not knowing what the reaction to my opening it might be. I never did do that (and now it appears my hesitation was onto something) but here I was ignoring my own caveat in pursuit of wanting input for this chapter.

I have written the above because I believe my experiences might very well be informative and helpful to colleagues. To restate: the conclusion I have reached is that successfully terminated long-term analyses, likely from any orientation, should not be reopened by the analyst for whatever reason short of announcements of extreme importance to the patient. It feels to me as if a boundary issue is involved that is difficult for me at this moment to clarify or even expand upon. Intrusion is the word used by one of my patients and intrusion is a word that cannot be understood without the concept of a boundary invasion.

It also occurs to me that there might be a kind of reawakening of a desire for the relationship with the analyst which has already been mourned and gotten beyond. If that's the case (and I believe that might very well be so) then contacting the patient includes a kind of tease, since no continuance is implied in the contact.

I realize there is much more to say about what happened and fully understand the patient who held back from opening this "psychoanalytic can of worms." But I could not ignore what happened and perhaps at some future time will focus more intently on the underlying dynamics of what occurred in an attempt to distinguish idiosyncratic responses from what might be generalizable – and therefore highly significant.

The person who agreed to write something for my first chapter and then again for this one, is currently seeing me once a month, and eight years ago was still in intensive treatment when I asked if she would like to add her thoughts to the chapter. Understandably, then, the issue of intrusion or reawakening had not arisen for her.

I want to add that in the midst of working on this chapter, I have begun to think that there might very well be other reasons for an analysis not ending, reasons having nothing to do with pathological dependence or fears of autonomy, but rather something else that needs to be respected for what it provides the patient, even if we are not sure what that might be. I realize these thoughts might constitute another paper. So at this point I'll just let them cook.

What follows are the comments from two patients. The first from the patient who stimulated my first paper and the second from the patient whom I asked if she would like to comment on her experiences leading up to, and subsequent to, the planned termination of her 11-and-a-half- year analysis. That patient is herself a psychoanalyst and writer and is the one who articulated ambivalent feelings about commenting.

First patient

> In my contribution to Dr. Glennon's earlier paper on Termination, I was clear that I wasn't prepared to take that that step. In reality I was quite prepared to end therapy. I simply wasn't prepared to terminate my relationship with Stefanie Glennon. In fact, I felt that to do so because of convention, would have called into question the authenticity of the rich and quite successful therapeutic journey we had, and the deep personal connection that played such a pivotal role in its success.
>
> In considering this dilemma, and after much discussion, we decided to try an experiment – break new ground if you will. I would terminate therapy but would come once a month, in an as yet nameless capacity, to catch up, visit and chat about whatever seemed to be present for both of us. For reasons which I believe will be obvious to each of you, it was decided I would pay my usual fee for the visit.
>
> That arrangement began on January 1, 2014 and continues to this day. In assessing, from my point of view, how it has worked, and noting it is still a work in progress, I would say this. I have gained much, and I have given up, and miss some appealing things.

Our relationship is much more relaxed, more casual and even more spontaneous. Most important to me is that the asymmetry, which had already diminished over time, is now even less and what remains is understandable.

What is proving harder to sustain is the day-to-day exchange and knowledge which comes from being together three times a week for many years. With that has come the lessening, not in the intensity of our connection, but in the immediacy of things that would have before been front and center.

As in all relationships there have been a few, very few I must say, hiccups along the way, but nothing to call this arrangement into question.

This new road we're on is I think, the best we can currently do in this situation, and with the same kind of care all relationships require in order to thrive, I believe it can and will go on quite nicely. One doesn't find very many deeply authentic and close relationships in life, and to my way of thinking, regardless of the circumstances in which they are born, they should be treasured and nurtured for as long as time allows.

Second patient

My reflections come with a caveat. Memories are colored by distance and one's current state of mind. Here is my conundrum: I don't entirely trust what I've written, yet I believe it's mostly true.

Devastated by the sudden death of our 23-year-old son, I began therapy in 1996. I could feel immediately Stefanie's capacity to hold me emotionally. She never flinched. I don't cry easily, but with her I wept freely, without fear of overwhelming her. She has a strong presence, and a desire to travel deeply into another's emotional experience. For a long time our focus was on my grief. Over the eleven years of our work, we also worked hard on my conflict about my aspirations. I had absorbed a belief that I was either a person who cared for others, or someone who was selfish. I was wary of "showing off." Our work enabled me to follow through with a newfound ambition to write a book about my grief process.

Within the first year of treatment, Stefanie told me that her husband was ill. Probably the context was her unexpected cancellations. I appreciated her honesty. She also let me know when he died. Some years later, Stefanie married an analyst whom I knew – in fact, he had referred me to her. When he suffered a catastrophic head injury in a bike accident three years later, Stefanie told me about it, and continued to update me, if I asked.

Shared grieving intensified our bond. But it wasn't the only reason for increased intimacy and affection between us. We liked each other, and I sensed that if we'd met as colleagues, we would have been friends. I didn't have that confidence right away. My old insecurities surfaced early in the transference. We worked on those, and on my family relationships. I had loving and sturdy bonds with my husband, two daughters and our sons-in-law, but our family was changed by our son's death. I grew, and learned, and engaged with life again, especially as our grandchildren came along.

After many years, I could more often anticipate Stefanie's responses to my material; I had taken in her voice, and largely integrated what I'd learned. As my storms of grief eased, writing provided another container for my sorrow. I still suffered from intermittent depression, a longstanding problem. I'd analyzed its conflict-driven aspects in a previous analysis, as well as with Stefanie. But depression is part of my family history, and our son's death had made me more susceptible to it. I kept it at bay with medication, which Stefanie hadn't encouraged, but she respected my decision.

I worried that leaving Stefanie could trigger a severe depression, as my retirement in 2003 had. But Stefanie would still be there. I'd spent years in therapy, and I wanted to be free of it. The WASP "do it yourself" model still lived in me. I began to resent paying to talk to someone whom I valued and loved, but whose wisdom and knowledge I'd mostly absorbed.

I remember asking, "Why would I *want* to leave you?" Psychoanalytic arguments were not persuasive. Why would internalization require separation? And surely I had learned that I could survive a traumatic loss. In light of our family's tragedy, I knew that mourning is never complete, but sorrow continues, living within us differently over time.

I understood psychoanalytic boundaries and didn't want a friendship. I wanted to hold Stefanie as a therapist who'd not only offered me extraordinary empathy and safety but had facilitated my creativity and agency. My "real relationship" with Stefanie had been forged in our shared experience of grief, and deepened by our analytic work. We shared a profession, as well as sensibilities and senses of humor. But most of our work was done, and I didn't want to be a patient anymore, or pay the fee. I felt more confident that a devoted husband, loving extended family, and intimate friends would sustain me.

In the end, I just had to gather the courage to say good-by. I was sad, but I was okay. I've been back for a few consultations, and Stefanie and I have occasionally been in touch by phone or email. Her life is challenging, and I want to know she's okay. But I have faith in her sturdiness. And my analysis – embedded in our relationship of depth, intimacy and love – has given me confidence in my own.

Afterword

I found the above comments to be extremely moving and affirming. Most significantly, I felt pride in both of these women, mainly for what they have accomplished in their lives, but also for their sensitivity, honesty, wisdom and articulateness. In addition there arose in me an unanticipated feeling, something akin to embarrassment insofar as the intimacy of our relationship was to some extent exposed. Not quite a breaking of confidentiality, but something similar. It is an interesting response on my part, but it certainly has not resulted in regret for having asked them to contribute to this chapter.

References

Bass, A. (2018). Discussant of "Being the change: Papers by Rachel Sopher and Kim Bernstein". IARPP Meetings, NYC.

Bergmann, M.S. (1997). Termination: The Achilles heel of psychoanalytic technique. *Psychoanalytic Psychology*, 14, 163–174.

Bollas, C. (1989). *The shadow of the object: Psychoanalysis of the unthought known*. New York: Columbia University Press.

Glennon, S.S. (2010). Relational analyses: Are they more difficult to terminate? In: Salberg, J. (ed.), *Good enough endings*. New York and Hove: Routledge, pp. 257–276.

Levenson, E.A. (1976). The aesthetics of termination. *Contemporary Psychoanalysis*, 12, 338–341.

Chapter 13

Neuropsychoanalysis and the repressed

Rendering what is possible in long-term psychotherapy

Jane Abrams

In 1975 Guntrip wrote of his analyses with Fairbairn and Winnicott. The title of his paper, "My Experience of Analysis with Fairbairn and Winnicott – (How Complete a Result Does Psycho-Analytic Therapy Achieve?)", poses a question that is among the many that we can ask ourselves when we reflect on long-term psychotherapy. In his paper Guntrip explained his understanding of why it wasn't until after 1,000 sessions with Fairbairn and 150 with Winnicott, and after both of these analysts had died, that he finally, through a dream, recovered a repressed memory of a childhood trauma that took place when he was 3 and a half years old – the sight of his dead baby brother on his mother's lap. He described the stark, though complementary, differences between the two analysts and how the work with each of them made it possible, eventually, for this memory to return to consciousness via the dream. He explained that, despite some negative maternal transference to Fairbairn, he had ultimately internalized Fairbairn as "another good father who had faith in me" (p. 155). Winnicott, he tells us, " … [entered] into the emptiness left by my non-relating mother, so that I could experience the security of being myself" (p. 155). He then went on to say:

> What is psychoanalytic psychotherapy? It is, as I see it, the provision of a reliable and understanding human relationship of a kind that makes contact with the deeply repressed traumatized child in a way that enables one to become steadily more able to live, in the security of a new relationship, with the traumatic legacy of the earliest formative years, as it seeps through or erupts into consciousness.
>
> (p. 155)

Guntrip was not using the language of relational theory or intersubjectivity, which was yet to come. However, he offered this quote from a session with Winnicott, in which Winnicott said to him:

> I'm good for you but you're good for me. Doing your analysis is almost the most reassuring thing that happens to me. The chap before you

> makes me feel I'm no good at all. You don't have to be good for me. I don't need it and can cope without it, but in fact you are good for me. (p. 153)

Here we are privy to Winnicott's reflections on how he was affected by Guntrip and how they cocreated a relationship that was positive for both of them. Guntrip (1975) described how Winnicott's joining with the deeply repressed, traumatized pre-oedipal child in him was mutative in a way that Fairbairn's more intellectualized interpretations, which were focused on oedipal dynamics, were not. Winnicott, as the internalized good object who "entered the emptiness" (p. 155) left by Guntrip's unresponsive mother, continued to hold him after the end of his analysis and even after Winnicott's death. The benefits of Guntrip's analysis with Winnicott endured and even increased over time. It is worth noting that among the results of Shedler's (2010) meta-analysis of studies measuring the efficacy of psychodynamic psychotherapies was the finding that patients who received psychodynamic therapy continued to benefit from underlying changes in their "intrapsychic processes" (p. 103) after treatment ended and symptoms had abated.

Guntrip's (1975) paper brings into focus some of the questions I would like to address: What is possible in psychodynamic therapy? What are the relational components, used in conjunction with what we are learning from neuropsychoanalysis about repression and the mechanics of memory, which make deep and lasting change possible? What is neuropsychoanalysis and how does it inform clinical practice? To assist in addressing these questions I will offer a case example of an ongoing enactment with one of my patients. I will use this case as an illustration of what is required of us relationally as we tangle with the repressed in a person who has experienced severe attachment trauma. I will then describe some of the central ideas in neuropsychoanalysis and how they might be helpful to clinicians engaged in long-term therapy relationships. I will conclude with personal reflections on the experience of being involved with patients over the course of many years.

Enactments

I am sure we can all relate to Winnicott's feelings of helplessness and badness with the "chap" he saw before his session with Guntrip, and with his relief of then seeing a patient with whom he felt connected and successful. Davies (2004) and Benjamin (2004, 2006) have provided us with examples of therapeutic impasses and a framework for understanding and navigating those times when we struggle with "being no good at all" (Guntrip, 1975, p. 153). It is these excruciating enactments, along with the less painful ones, which open up the possibility for deep change in our patients and for new learning about ourselves. As Davies (2004) has illustrated, one of the relational conditions that both opens the space for enactments to emerge and creates opportunities to grow from them is the therapist's capacity to deeply engage with the projections and projective identification within the therapeutic dyad. The therapist must do as Guntrip described – make contact with the traumatized child, whose suffering is expressed non-verbally.

Neuropsychoanalysis helps us understand why it might never be possible to remember the original trauma. However, its derivatives – maladaptive patterns of behavior and the accompanying feelings that repression cannot keep out of consciousness – are available for discovery and articulation in the holding environment of the therapy relationship. Therefore, the challenge of facilitating lasting change in our patients requires of us a deep and vulnerable engagement with the present-day attempts by our patients to find safety in an attachment. The greater their fear, the more confusing, hurtful, enraging, frustrating and, at times, unbearable their attempts at closeness to us will be – for them and for us. We must be willing to feel no good at all and then to try to understand what in our current interactions with our patient is evoking this feeling in us. We then have to be willing to face what it is that we are doing that is contributing to our patient also feeling no good at all.

Case example

Steven began treatment with me 15 years ago, when he was experiencing intense anxiety after beginning a new job. The first rupture in our relationship occurred a few months into his treatment and marked the beginning of an enactment that continues to the present day. When he experiences me as not understanding him, he lashes out verbally with a dissociated aggression that has, at times, evoked feelings in me of being punched and bruised. At those times, I am conscious of wanting to hurt him back. I have come to understand that, for Steven, being in a relationship means hurting and being hurt. This dynamic underlies the ongoing enactment in his treatment with me as well as in other relationships in his life. Although I know little about Steven's early life, I have observed from his present-day interactions with his mother that she is enmeshed with him in a most malignant way. She possesses a destructive negativity that has become part of who Steven is too – a self-state that murders all hope and agency.

Steven's father left the family when Steven was around 3 years old. He became "man of the house", feeling responsible for his mother's happiness. She did the best she could to care for her family – Steven and two younger siblings – but she never recovered from her husband's abandonment, which left her struggling financially, chronically angry and overwhelmed. In addition, Steven has hinted that she has a history of early childhood deprivation. What I have observed over the years between Steven and his mother is a pattern of her being agreeable and supportive of plans, goals and achievements in Steven's life, and then turning on him and attacking him with brutal, shaming criticism for his life choices. This leaves him not only devastatingly sad, but also enraged, helpless and hopeless. He can do nothing to please her, nothing he does is good enough and nothing in his life feels that it will have lasting value. He cannot trust himself to know whether what he does is worthwhile or whether he is safe in a given relationship. It is not simply that his mother is critical, but she attacks him with sadistic contempt, a part of her wanting to hurt him. She attempts to preserve her own sense of goodness by placing all the badness in him. That part of her has become part of him, a self-state that remains out of his conscious awareness. Steven and I do have peaceful periods that feel collaborative, when I feel that we have established a therapeutic alliance. At those times, I feel a deep fondness for him and a respect for his formidable talents. I can be the good mother and he can take in my affection and support. Then, out of the blue, he once again accuses me of utterly, completely failing him. Something in our interaction has caused him to panic. He attacks, becoming the punishing, hurting mother and I become the helpless, enraged, frightened child.

Several years ago, I immersed myself in Benjamin's work in the hopes of gaining a deeper understanding of what was driving the enactment with Steven. Her concepts of recognition, complementarity, the wounding healer and the failed witness have been particularly enlightening. Recognition (1995) – the ability of two people to understand each other, be attuned to each other, to perceive and relish the subjectivity of each other – describes what is missing between Steven and me when we are stuck in our impasses. According to Benjamin, mutual recognition is a developmental achievement that makes it possible for two people to experience each other as separate subjects, distinct from one another, yet able to fathom each other's minds. Complementarity (2004) is Benjamin's term for the relational dynamics that arise when recognition breaks down. During a therapeutic impasse, the ability of therapist and patient to experience each other as differentiated subjects degrades, and they become objects to each other, defined by each other's projections. The therapist becomes the "wounding healer" (Benjamin, 2006, p. 1), knowing she is hurting her patient, feeling shame, confused about where to place responsibility for the impasse and fearful of causing further harm. Below are some of my musings from that time when I was digging deeply into Benjamin's work. They illustrate my struggle with blame, responsibility, shame, fear of doing harm and how the concept of the failed witness helped me to recover some of my agency in the relationship:

> The reason that I cannot surrender to Steven's projections is that the nature of our complementarity is such that if I take on all the responsibility for our impasses and he takes on none of it, the good in me, my sense of self as a good person, will be destroyed. At those moments, I feel that all he sees are my failures. I know that this feeling is part of his experience too. I distance myself from him and that distancing is

> a further trigger for him. He senses immediately when I have shut down, which increases his panic, expressed as cruel aggression. While I can own my therapeutic mistakes, my moments of empathic failure, I cannot bear to have all my goodness erased.
>
> It helps me to know that according to Benjamin (2006), it would not be therapeutic for me to claim what is not mine in the enactment, to submit to Steven's demand that I take on all the badness, as his mother demands of him. Benjamin warned against the therapist's tendency towards self-blame. To take responsibility for what is not ours robs us of our agency. However, Steve cannot yet recognize his part in our impasses and still maintain his self-cohesion. For my part, I have not been able to make the space safe enough for him to do so. We remain in a stand-off of "doer and done to" (Benjamin, 2004, p. 5). At these times, we both feel erased. Russell (2006a) has told us that crises in treatment are in part communications from patients of feelings that they cannot put into words, but are compelled to act out. Treatment crises are opportunities for us to know what it is like to be them. This concept has been central to my practice since my training years, guiding me to use my countertransference as invaluable information about my patients, as well as about myself. However, it is still too frightening for Steven to be "known" and thus my attempts to connect with him around our shared experiences of failure, shame and helplessness in our relationship have not helped to free us from the doer and done to dynamic.

During this time, I consulted on Steven's case with a colleague who is an expert on dissociation. My colleague told me that there was indeed something I was not hearing. While I was describing Steven's treatment, my colleague could hear a child crying out to a mother who wouldn't hear him. I felt relieved to have gained conscious awareness of this self-state of Steven's. At the same time, I felt shame over having missed this and having hurt Steven by not hearing him. I needed to understand what was going on within me and between us that was getting in the way of my hearing this child's voice. Eventually I realized that I share a self-state with Steven – that of the child who is trying her best but whose good intentions are met with criticism and shaming. When Steven lashes out at me and doesn't recognize my earnest attempts to help him, he becomes my bad object and I withdraw in an attempt to regulate my own shame and rage.

Benjamin's concept of the failed witness (2004) eased my guilt and shame about not hearing the crying child. I could accept not always being a perfect listener. What I had been unable and unwilling to do was to submit to Steven's demand that I take on the role of the one who has failed completely and furthermore, wants to and has intentionally hurt him. With some distance from these projections I was able to more freely explore what it was that I didn't want to hear and why. I became aware of how hard it is for me to sit with Steven's hopelessness and destructiveness. I find it unbearable when he destroys not just all the goodness between us but all the goodness in his life. I resist his assault on hope. He erases himself and all his talents, his generosity, his accomplishments. I feel angry, not at him or at myself, but at the psychological legacy in Steven's family that now makes it so hard for him to recognize himself, to appreciate himself and to have empathy for himself.

The oscillations between recognition and complementarity in my work with Steven have been exhausting. I have not always welcomed the intense self-examination that has been required of me in order stay fully engaged with him. It certainly helps to have this process normalized by these words from Benjamin:

> There may be no tenet more important to overcoming this shame and blame in analytic work than the idea that recognition continually breaks down, that thirdness always collapses into twoness, that we are always losing and recovering the intersubjective view.
>
> (2004, p. 29)

What is neuropsychoanalysis and can it help?

Psychoanalytic theory offers many conceptual frameworks for understanding the kind of repetition that is playing out in the enactments between Steven and me, such as the repetition compulsion, the internalization of our early relationships, dissociative processes and the defense mechanisms of repression, projection, projective identification and splitting. As I have become familiar with discoveries in neuroscience, especially those regarding the dynamics of memory, I have found that they provide new explanations for my lived experience with my patients while validating the psychoanalytic theories that have guided me throughout my career. It is no surprise that I am drawn, therefore, to neuropsychoanalysis. Neuropsychoanalysis is an interdisciplinary field founded by Mark Solms in the 1980s and based on the premise that integrating the findings of neuroscience and the psychoanalytic model of the mind will result in a deeper understanding of mental life. One of the current goals of the field is to encourage and bring together the work of neuroscientists who think psychodynamically and can contribute research that establishes a neuroscientific basis for psychoanalytic theory and practice. For psychodynamic ideas and practice to survive in today's world, we need this science. We need to be able to counter perceptions that what we do is somehow "faith-based" (Schwartz, 2015, paragraph 5). Neuropsychoanalysis is concerned largely with the biological substrates of affects, the parameters of consciousness and the dynamics of memory and repression (Solms, 2013,

2017b). The clinical application of neuropschoanalytic findings is an area still in its infancy and one which I will explore in this chapter. First, I will summarize some of the key ideas in neuropsychoanalysis that I think are applicable to our work, especially to long-term treatment.

Affective neuroscience is a branch of the neurosciences that is central to neuropsychoanalysis. The late Jaak Panskepp is credited with creating a taxonomy of seven basic affective systems located in the subcortical region of the brain, the upper brain stem, which are shared by all mammals and some vertebrates (Panskepp & Biven, 2012). These systems are: the Seeking System, which leads us out into the world not only to get our needs met but to satisfy our innate curiosity, the Panic/Grief System, activated during separations from caregivers, the Care System, our need to nurture and care for others, especially our offspring, the Lust System, the need for sexual partners, ensuring procreation, the Fear System, the need to escape dangerous situations, the Rage System, our response to frustration, and the Play System, the need for the rehearsal of the establishment of social hierarchies. Panskepp labeled these seven systems as our "homeostatic affects". Solms (2017b) referred to these as our "need detectors" (p. 92), each with feelings attached to them. Panskepp referred to these as the "universal affective mind" (p. 7). The more complex human emotions involve learning and thought and are affected by culture and the environment. These include empathy, trust, blame, pride, guilt, shame, and disgust, among others. Our homeostatic affects – our need detectors – reside in our primary process emotional systems.

Solms (2017a) asserted that the main task of development is to figure out how to get our needs met; needs that arise from the activation of these seven basic affective systems. He went on to say that the reason that life is hard is that we need other people to meet these needs. Here is where learning and memory come into play. Each one of us must figure out how to get our needs met in the environments we are born into. As we know only too well, this often means that children have to make the best of bad situations. Solms (2017b) asserted that the work of the ego is to figure out how to get our needs met and how to manage the feelings that are attached to these needs. We seek quiescence – the absence of needs, which only comes when our needs are satisfied.

The ego makes predictions regarding how to get needs met in the world (Solms, 2017b). These predictions become what Solms referred to as action plans. Sometimes a child is faced with the impossibility of getting certain of her needs met, an insoluble problem, and must devise a plan that involves compromise. Her action plan represents the best that she can do, a work-around, if you will, of the insoluble problem. These action plans become deeply automatized, or repressed. Because they are compromises that don't completely solve the problem, they do not manage all the feelings that are connected to the unmet needs. Thus, the need for secondary defenses arises. We no longer have conscious access to the compromise action plan, or the trauma that necessitated it, but the feelings are consciously accessible. As Solms (2017a) stated, "psychological patients suffer mainly from feelings" (p. 4).

The reason that our action plans remain unconscious has to do with how memory works. In fact, only 5% of our goal-directed behaviors are conscious (Bargh & Chartrand, 1999). Our action plans are put into place very early in childhood, before the areas of the brain necessary for the formation of explicit or declarative memory have matured. They are stored in the brain as implicit or non-declarative memories – they have bypassed thinking. Another type of implicit or non-declarative memory is procedural memory. These are our memories of how to perform certain tasks, formed by repeating a complex activity over and over again to establish the neural networks that can automatically produce the action. Through a process called consolidation, these non-verbal, non-thinkable memories become deeply unconscious (Milekic & Alberini, 2002). To change a long-term memory, it has to come into consciousness again and then become reconsolidated – returned, in its revised form, to long-term memory storage. Solms (2017b) stated that the implicit nature of repressed action plans means that they are indelible, forever repressed. A non-declarative memory is forever unthinkable.

If we can never retrieve these memories, if they are forever unthinkable and unrevisable, then where does that leave us with our patients? We can infer the nature of the original action plan by its derivatives – the patterns repeating in a person's life and the feelings associated with the patterns. We can help our patients think about how their action plans are, in their present lives, not working and help them embrace the possibility of formulating new action plans. "What patients *can* think about – can problematize, if it is brought to their attention – is the repetitive *derivatives* of the repressed" (Solms, 2017b, p. 95). We work with the feelings that were unsuccessfully managed by the early, compromise action plan. The feelings assist us and our patients in identifying needs that are not being met.

Therapeutic impasses and enactments

Solms (2017b) referred to uncertainty that arises when the ego perceives a prediction error. This uncertainty is an arousal state that signals that an action plan is not working and needs to be updated. I suggest that it is this uncertainty that can cause therapeutic impasses and prolonged enactments, like the one I am involved in with Steven. This is where relational theory, intersubjectivity and the mutative potential of the therapist–patient relationship can inform neuropsychoanalysis about the therapeutic conditions that are necessary for the revision of action plans that are not working. There has to be enough trust and holding in the therapeutic relationship for our patients to be able to tolerate the uncertainty of deep change. They are not going to give up a familiar way of being for a totally new way of being unless they *feel held* during the transition.

I think about what it's like to teach a child to ride a bicycle. The ability to ride a bike eventually becomes an unconscious, procedural memory. You practice until the neural networks are created that make it possible for you ride a bike, and then it becomes a memory that is no longer thinkable. It becomes an automatic action. However, children need a great deal of support during the uncertain phase when they want to give up their training wheels but don't know how to stay upright on a two-wheeler. They need a parent to support them physically, holding on to the back of their seat, so that when they lose their balance they won't get seriously hurt. They need their parent to hold onto the hope and the certainty that they will master this task and that life will be better when they can zip around on their own. They need to trust that their parent will know when to hold on and when to let go. As we know, building this level of trust can take some of our patients a very long time.

Action plans or the repetition compulsion?

How is the concept of action plans or predictions different from Freud's concept of the repetition compulsion? In terms of what comprises the contents of the repressed, I do not think there is a difference. However, there is a powerful difference in the language when comparing these terms; the compulsion to repeat versus an action plan that no longer works. The latter more strongly suggests a sense of agency and the potential for change. It can be shame-reducing to explain to a patient that what he did was to try to make the best of a bad situation, to solve an insoluble problem, but now that strategy isn't working so well. Furthermore, understanding the biology of memory and repression provides a neuroscientific understanding for why we get stuck in old patterns, and also why there is always the potential for change.

MacDuffie and Strauman (2017) have introduced the term "auto-biology" to describe biological information given to people suffering from psychiatric disorders whose origins are considered to be biological, such as some types of depression. They suggest a framework that delivers a message that will increase the likelihood that patients will use information about their biology in a way that increases self-efficacy – what you are suffering from is not your fault and you can change it. Biological systems are not static, but dynamic and ever-changing. MacDuffie and Strauman consider this a prospective framing – a focus on how patients can cope with and improve their systems, rather than feel that they are destined to suffer due to their biology. "The overarching message that should be communicated in a prospective biological frame is that experience can change the brain. Indeed, one could go even further and argue that brains are 'designed' to be responsive to experience" (p. 60).

Neuropsychoanalysis offers biological explanations for the nature and origins of our needs, how we adapted to our environments, what has happened to our earliest memories, how and why memories remain inaccessible, how we might gain access to some of them and how we can benefit from that access. Neuropsychoanalysis provides evidence that both nature and nurture make us who we are. It tells us that there are certain needs and feelings that we share not just with all humans but with all other mammals and some birds as well. At the same time, each of is born into a family, a culture, a socioeconomic situation that demands that we adapt as best we can. For many, this involves compromises that can cause much suffering. Using a neuropsychoanalytic perspective, I can help Steven see that he is not an utter failure, but that he succeeded at adapting to his environment the best way he could, finding ways to satisfy as many of his basic needs as possible. This is a strengths-based message and one which reflects social work's long-held biopsychosocial view of the human mind. It demonstrates the potential for Steven to formulate a new action plan that will result in more of his needs being met in his current environment. The incubator for this new plan is the therapeutic relationship.

Steven's action plan

Steven sometimes lets me be the parent holding onto his bike seat while he works on the coordination necessary for him to keep his balance on his own. But then I let go too soon, or push too hard, or fail to notice how frightened he is, and he gives up on me. He reverts back to his tried and true action plan: "I guess I'm on my own because there is no one available who can help me. The ones who are supposed to help me always let me down and hurt me. So, I have to do it myself". I need to keep working on what in our intersubjective space makes it impossible most of the time for me to make contact with that child who has not been heard. What parts of my action plan map onto his, contributing to our stubborn impasses? For now, with Steven, I am more like Fairbairn in Guntrip's treatment than I am like Winnicott. I have not found a way to enter into the deeply traumatized parts of him in a way that will facilitate healing. I hold back, as Fairbairn did. For Steven's part, letting go of his old action plan and implementing a new one is still terrifying. If I hear him, he is no longer alone. However, since he is still not ready to give up the safety of aloneness, he continues to make it hard for me to hear him. He is not ready yet for "the safety of aloneness [to be] gradually, very slowly, relinquished in favor of an utterly new event: safety within a relationship" (Russell, 2006b, p. 44).

Since our repressed action plans, or predictions, are never available to consciousness and thus revision, they are always with us, existing alongside any new action plans that have been formulated in long-term therapy. Therefore Steven, like Guntrip, will always, to some extent, be haunted by his early attachment trauma. However, if Steven discovers the benefits of closeness to people who do not want to hurt him (and builds the confidence that he can recognize who is safe and who is not), I hope that, over time, he will be able to formulate and embrace a new action plan that includes the possibility of being safe in relationships. Perhaps one day he will be able to recognize fragments of the old action plan as they arise – "seep through" (Guntrip, 1975, p. 155) – and identify them as vestiges of a strategy for survival that was once the best he could do but has become ineffective and self-defeating in his present life. Perhaps he will be able to free himself from the constraints of the fearful, hyperviligant, self-protectively aggressive space that he inhabits and then move with greater joy through the world.

Reflections on the experience of the therapist

Like my work with Steven, some long-term treatments are characterized by disorienting and painful enactments. I doubt that any of us could sustain our careers as therapists over the decades were it not for the many patients with whom the ongoing work is less volatile and involves a process more akin to Tronick's (1989) description of the cycles of attunement, disruption and repair that are the unconscious, intersubjective, rhythmic underpinnings of healthy development. When ruptures are less severe and ongoing repairs occur, both therapist and patient have the freedom and confidence to continually take risks in the service of deeper intimacy and self-knowledge.

Russell (2006b) reminded us of our responsibility to remain committed to believing in the ongoing possibility of change in our patients.

> As long as there is life and living there is the potential for further healing and growth. It seems to me that what one does in the treatment situation is to provide an environment as optimal as possible for the healing process to occur, and to allow [it to] evolve at will.
>
> (p. 11)

I would add that, in order to do this, we must remain equally committed to our own growth and guard against complacency in ourselves as well as in our work with patients. Moreover, the self- knowledge I am gaining in my work with Steven benefits all my patients and, indeed, all of my relationships.

The hard and painful work that can characterize some long-term treatment relationships is balanced by the intensely pleasurable feelings of connection, affection, and familiarity that I experience with most of my long-term patients. As we greet each other at the beginning of each session and sit down in our customary places in my office to resume our work, we pick up where we left off – a week ago, a month ago, sometimes several years ago. My patients are the beneficiaries of my unique knowledge of them and of the holding environment that, over the years, they have come to rely on. They know that I keep them in mind. I am a beneficiary of the intimacy we share and of the privilege they grant me of bearing witness to parts of themselves that, for many, they have revealed for the first time to me. I travel with them through their lives, participating in their healing and their triumphs and sharing their losses. I benefit from the continuing challenge to become a better listener, to dig deeper into my own mind to discover the barriers in me that compromise my ability to hear certain kinds of pain. My work with Steven, in particular, has pushed me to grow in these ways. I join with other writers who have described the trust that we build with our patients as sacred and with those writers who strive for the words to describe this most unusual relationship. For example, Lord (2008) offered the following reflections:

> Therapeutic interactions take place in relationships that evolve over time within the disciplined parameters of an environment that is what I think of as a mutually cultivated sacred space. The dimensions of therapeutic relationships, including time limits, boundaries, and ethical behaviors required, exist to promote safety and the development of trust. These parameters take the relationships out of time and space and make them, I would venture to say, more real and more unreal than just about any other possible human interaction.
>
> (p. 120)

These "more real and more unreal" relationships enrich our lives in ways so numerous and complex that we could fill multiple volumes describing them.

Analysis terminable?

Now that I am getting older, I have begun to hear comments from patients like, "We are growing old together" and "I still have lots of work to do. I hope that you have no plans to retire any time soon". I think of Guntrip and Fairbairn. Guntrip (1975) described Fairbairn as past his creative prime as a theoretician and clinician when he entered analysis with him. When Fairbairn suffered a near-fatal illness and became, in the transference, Guntrip's dead brother Percy, Guntrip felt that Fairbairn was too frail to engage with him in analyzing this new dimension of his transference.

Steven needs continuing deep engagement from me. There are days when it seems that he is inching his way towards being able to trust that I am on his side, despite my lapses. I think of Fairbairn and Guntrip and hope that I will have the stamina to continue this often grueling work for as long as it takes. I want to guard against retreating to a theoretical or clinical stance that feels safe and familiar to me but misses what it is that Steven needs from me, as Fairbairn apparently did by rigidly adhering to his oedipal interpretations of Guntrip's pre-oedipal attachment trauma (Guntrip, 1975).

Relational principles remain a steadfast guide, as does Russell's (2006b) admonition to remain committed to the possibility of growth and healing across the lifespan – ours and our patients'. Emerging scientific explanations of the workings of memory and repression can help light the way when a confusion of past with present (ours and our patients') threatens the survival of the therapy relationship. If I were to answer Guntrip's (1975) question, posed in the title of his paper – "How Complete a Result Does Psycho-Analytic Therapy Achieve?" – I would have to say it depends on the particular patient working with a particular therapist. Perhaps it boils down to how resilient each of them is. To what extent can each tolerate the uncertainty of change? How flexible is the intersubjective space that exists at the intersection of the action plans of therapist and patient? Did each experience enough attachment security so that the repair of ruptures is a possibility? It takes time to discover how much potential for change each patient possesses. This is one of the unknowns we embrace with each new referral. For our part, we can work throughout our lives on our own healing and towards deeper self-knowledge so that we can optimize the possibilities for growth for our patients.

References

Bargh, J., & Chartrand, T. L. (1999). The unbearable automaticity of being. *American Psychologist*, *54*, 462–479.

Benjamin, J. (1995). Recognition and destruction: An outline of intersubjectivity. In *Like subjects, love objects: Essays on recognition and sexual difference*, pp. 27–48. New Haven, CT: Yale University Press.

Benjamin, J. (2004). Beyond doer and done to. *Psychoanalytic Quarterly*, *73(1)*, 5–46.

Benjamin, J. (2006, January). *Our appointment in Thebes: Acknowledgment, the failed witness and the analyst's fear of harming*. Paper presented at the annual meeting of the International Association for Relational Psychoanalysis, Boston, MA.

Davies, J. M. (2004). Whose bad objects are we anyway? Repetition and our elusive love affair with evil. *Psychoanalytic Dialogues*, *14*, 711–732.

Guntrip, H. (1975). My experience of analysis with Fairbairn and Winnicott – (how complete a result does psycho-analytic therapy achieve?). *International Review of Psycho-Analysis*, *2*, 145–156.

Lord, S. A. (2008). Therapeutic work with trauma, revictimization, and perpetration: Bearing witness, offering hope, embracing despair. *Psychoanalytic Social Work*, *15*, 110–131.

MacDuffie, K., & Strauman, T. (2017). Understanding our own biology: The relevance of auto-biological attributions for mental health. *Clinical Psychology Science and Practice*, *24*, 50–68.

Milekic, M., & Alberini, C. (2002). Temporally graded requirement for protein synthesis following memory reactivation. *Neuron*, *36*, 521–525.

Panskepp, J., & Biven, L. (2012). *The archaeology of mind: Neuroevolutionary origins of human emotions*. New York, NY: W. W. Norton & Company.

Russell, P. (2006a). The theory of the crunch. *Smith College Studies in Social Work*, *76*, 9–21.
Russell, P. (2006b). The compulsion to repeat. *Smith College Studies in Social Work*, *76*, 33–49.
Schwartz, C. (2015, June 28). Tell it about your mother. Retrieved from: https://www.nytimes.com/2015/06/28/magazine/tell-it-about-your-mother.html?ref=magazine.
Shedler, J. (2010). The efficacy of psychodynamic psychotherapy. *American Psychologist*, *65*, 98–109.
Solms, M. (2013). The conscious id. *Neuropsychoanalysis*, *15*, 5–19.
Solms, M. (2017a, January). *The scientific standing of psychoanalysis.* Paper presented at the meeting of American Psychoanalytic Association, New York, NY.
Solms, M. (2017b). What is "the unconscious", and where is it located in the brain? A neuropsychoanalytic perspective. *Annals of the New York Academy of Sciences*, *1406*, 90–96.
Tronick, E. Z. (1989). Emotions and emotional communication in infants. *American Psychologist*, *44*, 112–119.

Chapter 14

The longest goodbyes

Analysis everlasting

Anthony Bass

The longest running analysis ever?

In Woody Allen's satirical version of psychoanalysis, the relationship between a patient and therapist may transcend the limits of life itself, for better or worse. A patient (Allen's comedic character Alvy Singer in *Annie Hall*) contemplates his elective departure from his mortal coil. Except for one thing. He is in analysis with a strict Freudian, and in therapy like that, the deal is that if you kill yourself while under care, you have to keep paying for all the sessions that you miss. So, he thinks better of it, galled (and maybe reassured) by the recognition (fantasy) that the analytic frame will remain securely in place, the bills for services rendered coming right on time as per the agreement, for eternity.

> If my analyst will persist in her labors behind the couch with or without me, perhaps I will stick around to reap the benefits of whatever improved mental health I might yet accrue, notwithstanding the discouraging results I have achieved thus far.

His thoughts of suicide might suggest to the layman that things haven't been going all that well so far, but as therapists and patients we know that both hope and dread, optimism and discouragement, love and hate, even life and death, are our constant companions in psychoanalysis.

In Allen's version of classical analysis, the analyst doesn't really say all that much anyway, so the long silences anticipated in a post-suicide world of treatment, though extreme, wouldn't be altogether unprecedented either. It seems that for Allen's character, avoiding the indignity of paying for 'missed sessions' would be as good a reason as any to stick around. 'I'll be damned if I'll pay that son of a bitch when he couldn't even keep me alive. I think I'll just stick around and have him earn his fee.' Jokes, like dreams, provide excellent pathways to 'the royal road on-ramps' to the unconscious that psychoanalysis paves for an exploration of patients' conscious and almost-conscious experience. So being an analyst who can also see the humor in what is serious doesn't hurt.

In that sense, analysis begins but never ends as an internal process because the relationship itself transcends ordinary bounds. Psychic reality is its truest currency, a place for dreams and fantasy to express and to illuminate inner life. Patients have 'conversations in their minds' with their therapists between sessions, on vacations, after analysis has ended, and after their analyst is no longer living. We carry our analysts' (past and present) voices with us, as 'good objects' and bad. Having worked with several analysts myself over many years I can easily conjure their distinct voices, some helpful, others harmful, as I can invoke my parents, old friends, patients past and present, and others who have had an impact on how I feel and think about myself. An analyst's voice is often a lifelong companion, for better or worse, but that voice can take many years to be 'fully vested,' to gain the traction of 'internal objects' that have established themselves before, and that color the patient's experience of new voices as well. When it does, it remains a significant voice in the internal chorus for the patient who carries it forward.

The voices we carry

A patient in her fourth year of analysis was talking about the damaging effects of a long-term marriage and the ways that our conversations were beginning to ease the sense of shame and anger that the marriage left her with. She said, perhaps with conscious hyperbole but I think also with some unconscious longing, that it would take her eighteen years of analysis to get over the traumatic effects of an eighteen-year marriage. Was she experiencing her therapy as the second marriage that might repair the first? And what of those first eighteen years of her life that prepared her for that choice of husband? Could the analyst's voice help her do battle with these as well? We have had a good start on this project of reclamation and restoration of herself, but the eighteen years she feels it will take to heal suggest we have a long way to go to counteract the shame and gaslighting that characterized her marriage and much of the life that preceded it as well.

The voices we carry are not always salutary, and analyst's voices are no exception. Analyses leave residues, good and bad. My patient, who had an extremely painful damaging first analysis, had a panic attack when she received an invitation to a party and saw that analyst's name on the e-invitation rsvp list. She had been looking forward to the party, but now she found to her chagrin that she could not go. She was troubled and confused that her friend could invite such a person to her party. It felt like a betrayal, however irrational she knew that was. She felt that to go to the party, to see him, would evoke the same pain, anger and shame with which she had left the analysis with him twenty years earlier. New memories from within that therapy emerged, new pieces of the puzzle that would help us to see what had gone wrong, and how she had participated in shaping the bad experience that she had had. She had finally been able to extricate herself from the analysis that had felt like quicksand when, returning to the waiting room from the restroom after a session, she heard her analyst greet his next patient with welcoming warmth, a sound she had not heard from him in their years together. She realized at that moment that she was right, that the analyst **really didn't like her**, that is was not a matter of the **transference** that her analyst insisted it was when she wondered about the source of what she felt was the analyst's icy distaste for her. She was amazed that the feelings were still so alive after all these years. It had taken fifteen years of 'recovery' to get over that experience enough to make another try in analysis with me. She told me that she knew by our third session that this would be a different experience, that she could hear it in the warmth of my voice. She wished she had been ready to give therapy another try sooner than she had. The years that had passed took her from age 32 to 47. She felt she had missed out on a lot in between that she now felt therapy might have made possible.

Once an analysis begins, it is impossible to say when it will end. Sometimes long analyses come in fits and starts, as patients come, go and return. I began working with a patient who contacted me by e-mail last summer while I was on vacation. 'You might not remember me,' the note said.

> I was your patient some time ago, and I would like to resume therapy if at all possible. I gather from what I see on the internet that you are still in practice, as I had hoped. I thought it was possible that you had retired. If you are available and able to resume our work, I would be very pleased.

I was disconcerted that I could not conjure the slightest trace of an image of the man who had held me firmly in mind all this time, and I must admit to the passing thought that this was a case of mistaken identity. Might he be seeking a different Dr. Bass? Would he show up at the appointed hour to find a stranger, to say, 'never mind, I am looking for a different Dr.'? Could he be searching for the **other** Dr. A. Bass in town whose mail I sometimes receive? Once, when giving a talk, someone in the audience commented on how much my work had changed since an article I had written twenty years earlier. The article, I explained to the laughter of the audience, was written by the other Dr. A. Bass.

In my return e-mail, I told him when I would be back from vacation, and that I could arrange a consultation then, adding, perhaps too casually to hide my anxious concern at my faulty memory and to convince myself that he had the right man, 'by the way, can you remind me when we last met?' 'Yes, it was twenty- five years ago,' he responded right away. 'I was 27 years old. I saw you for a year in my last year of medical school. I stopped when I finished and went on to residency.' He was beginning to come back to me now; it was a therapy that never seemed to quite take off.

> You have been on my mind quite a lot since then, as I knew that I had not been altogether honest with you about some of my problems, which have been plaguing me ever since. Things have gotten quite bad in the last few years, with a marriage and other things that have gotten out of hand, and I have often thought that had I been able to be more honest with you then, you could have been more helpful. I wasn't honest with myself either. I wonder if I might have been able to head off some of the problems that I am dealing with now.

I would learn some months later, once our analysis had resumed, that there was a part of the patient that felt 'I should have known better,' wishing that I had had what it would have taken to see through the façade that had apparently lulled us both so unfortunately to sleep. I could have known that there was more to him than met my eye (I?).

But that conversation would come later. I realized in thinking about his initial messages that initiated the second phase of his analysis with me that I have vivid, distinct memories of several patients that I had known early in my practice. They have occupied my mind in various ways since our parting, like friends with whom I have fallen out of touch. I wonder how his life has been, how the children have grown up, whether her mother is still alive. Now, I could have wondered whether this kind of memory had gone missing with him partly because of an elusiveness I must have sensed at the time (had he ever really been there?).

But the other part I recognized was my inability as a young analyst to 'find him,' or to find him in myself. This, I now realized, left me disconnected from him, and perhaps more importantly, from myself. Had I ever truly been there with him? I was glad to have another chance to find out whether we could make more of his analysis now, with twenty-five years more of practice under my belt. I sometimes wish that patients with whom I struggled would return, thinking that I could help them more now because of all I have learned since, and what I learned from failing with them. In this case, I would have a chance to test that theory. I was grateful for the chance. And so we resumed an 'analysis interruptus' after a twenty-five year hiatus.

In the Allen image, the denial of death (another of Allen's central themes) and the seeming impossibility of actually ending an analysis become reassuringly one. If Woody Allen's joke had been written prior to Freud's 'Jokes and their Relation to the Unconscious' (1953), Freud might have employed it as a good example of what jokes can accomplish in their mining and linking of dense and surprising unconscious connections with the salve of a laugh—in this case about endings (of life and analysis), as well as other universal themes: money, power dynamics, separations and more. In another joke, offering another comedic take on the interminability, in one lifetime, of an analysis, from his movie *Sleeper*, his character wakes up after 200 years in a cryogenic coma, which he entered in the first place in an effort to cheat death. Among his first comments upon awakening is 'I haven't seen my analyst in 200 years. He's a strict Freudian. If I had still been going, I'd be almost cured by now.'

I believe that Allen's joke captures an essential truth of analysis. Were we to live for 250 years, there would be more to say, more to know, and more that would remain unknowable. Indeed, psychoanalysis is often a very lengthy process, its ultimate duration indeterminate. An analysis might turn out to be brief; it might last a lifetime. A patient phoned for a consultation today, leaving a message with some questions, including how long therapy would likely take. Some version of this question is not unusual. I typically say something like 'I don't know, it will depend on how helpful you find it to be, and how far you would like to take it.' There is no definitive stopping point limned with a robotic GPS voice that says, 'you have arrived at your destination.' In psychoanalysis, the route and destination are always 'recalculating' as the relationship between therapist and patient deepens, and more is experienced and discovered.

A patient's sense of how long an analysis might go may be clearer at the beginning of analysis than at any time before saying goodbye, because s(he) begins with conscious intentions and misconceptions about (her)himself and the process, which experience and what the unconscious makes of it will repeatedly disrupt and recontextualize along the way. Only the psychoanalytic explorations that follow will be informative about what the patient needs, wants, and how far the analytic couple will find it is possible to go, 'for the time being.'

Sacks: beginning to get somewhere now

Oliver Sacks, the essayist, memoirist and neurologist, spoke about his own experience in psychoanalysis as it evolved from an acute, critical emergency to a meandering process of personal growth and enrichment over many decades. He described it this way well into its fourth decade in a 2011 interview conducted for *Web of Stories*:

> I was dangerously drug-addicted at that time. I was taking huge doses of amphetamines on the weekends, potentially fatal doses. I specialized in overdoses. On the last day of the year, 1965, I had lost 65 or 70 pounds in a few months. I had a sober moment. 'Oliver,' I said, 'you will not see another New Year's Day, unless you get help.' So I took myself along to a psychoanalyst … I have been seeing Dr. Shengold for a little more than 46 years. I saw him this morning. I am speaking in 2011. I first saw him in 1966. *No doubt, this is one of the longest analyses on record. At least I like to think so. I think also that we are beginning to get somewhere now* (emphasis mine). Dr. Shengold and I have grown old together. We've gone through life stages together.
>
> (Sacks, 2011)

Sacks would die four years after completing this interview, from cancer. I expect that Sacks and his analyst had fifty years together by the end, living through life's trials and celebrations as each of them evolved and lived a full life from young manhood to old age (Leonard Shengold is 92 years old, and continues to practice in NYC).

Growing old together is indeed the fate of each analytic couple who stays the course of analysis over decades

To the uninitiated (those not knowing psychoanalysis from the inside out as patient and/or therapist), and to young analysts and patients too young to have experienced such sweeps of life, Sacks' remark that *he is beginning to get somewhere now* (after forty-six years!) might raise an eyebrow. Even I, an analyst of thirty-five years' experience currently working with at least two patients for over thirty years (and several others more than twenty), gave over to a chuckle in hearing Sack's sanguine observation (*I am beginning to get somewhere now*) about a life (two lives) spent together in therapy. It wasn't the sardonic, ambivalent chuckle of Allen's satire (I might be almost—but not quite—finished if I had been seeing my analyst for the whole 200 years). Rather my response combined a sense of recognition (of my own decades-long relationships in analysis as both therapist and patient), and amazement at the ways in which any given analytic relationship has the potential to deepen and to enrich lives through the decades. Most analysts would I think resonate with Sack's observation that he is 'finally getting someplace.' An 80-year-old training analyst that I know noted that it is unfortunate that the American Psychoanalytic Association has a rule against taking on a training analysis past the age of 70. 'I am finally getting the hang of this, it takes a long time you know,' he said with a twinkle in his eye. Another working analyst in his 90s, a former teacher and supervisor of mine, and now a favorite lunch companion, told me recently over our sushi that he is still excited about what he is learning from his patients. He is getting better at his job, and so he is glad that he is now 'too old to retire.'

Since analysts learn about themselves throughout their careers by doing the work, and learn more about themselves from each encounter with a patient, the learning curve for an analyst often continues for a lifetime. I believe that this is one of the reasons that few analysts actually retire; it is hard to give up a process when one is still learning from it. And it is also one of the reasons why patients stay in analysis as long as they do.

Sack's observation about the joint negotiation of life's challenges is a familiar trope. I have worked with patients who have known me as I have gotten married, become a father, lost parents, worried about my children, lived through my own and my family's illnesses, had children graduate from high school and college, and so on. And I have known my patients through all such life transitions, and more as well. It is not that each patient knows the details of our lives, but they see, learn and intuit a lot. They notice that wedding rings appear on their therapist's finger, and that they sometimes disappear. A patient told me in my first year of private practice that she realized that my wife had had a miscarriage. Stunned, I asked her how she had known.

> Well, you seemed up and quite excited for a while a few months after I noticed your new ring. Then you came in looking pale, not well, deflated. I worried about you. I felt that your wife must have lost a baby, but I didn't want to invade your privacy, so I didn't mention it, until now when I can see you are feeling better. Are you expecting another child?

We were.

Each partner in therapy becomes invested over time in the well-being and growth of the other. My patients have seen me grow, change and struggle over the years, as I have seen them. When patients do end therapy, especially after many years, they often say something in recognition of how I have changed too, and how they believe they have contributed to the changes they have seen in me. And how my changing has helped them to grow too. In any analysis worth its salt, both participants change as a function of their encounter with one another, and it is helpful for that to be recognized, appreciated and celebrated. I believe I have been helpful to my own analysts, and they have said as much, except for one, who didn't help me either. The mutuality of the psychoanalytic relationship is such that each partner is invested in the growth of the other, because each person's growth both relies and furthers the growth of the other.

Though most therapists who have been in practice long enough have at least a patient or two that they have seen for more than a couple of decades, I find that therapists and patients alike sometimes suffer from ambivalence, even guilt, about such long-term work.

> Am I doing this well? Is this analysis going on for too long? Should I be better at helping my patient to separate? If so, what is in the way of that and what am I contributing to the difficulty? Am I holding on to the patient because of my own needs and self -interests, more than theirs?

One source of such concern may be that many therapists have relatively little experience bringing analyses to a close. Since most analyses take longer to complete than does analytic training itself, few analysts have any experience of 'terminating' analysis while in training. Even later in careers, it is unusual for an analyst to end with more than one or two patients a year (Balint, 1950). As a result, most analysts have more confidence in their abilities to be helpful in the midst of an analysis than in helping a patient to end it, which can add a degree of insecurity, and even shame, when it comes to negotiating the late stages of an analysis. A pilot or copilot who is better at flying than landing the plane will suffer appropriate anxiety as the destination nears. I recall an early supervisor of mine who referred to some patients as 'lifers,' and another who opined that each analytic therapist has within their practice a 'chronic ward.' 'Lifers,' of course, carries the connotation of imprisonment for high crimes, and 'a chronic ward' evokes images of severely impaired psychiatric patients who need lifelong care with little expectation of meaningful improvement of their lot.

Although there are undoubtedly patients who rely on long-term work as a kind of maintenance in the service of physical and psychological survival, this does not reflect my typical experience of work that persists for many years. When it does, it is usually more complicated than such an image suggests. A patient of mine who I have been seeing for twenty-five years, recently said that she doesn't know what she would do without me (what if I die?). I began seeing her early in her career, and she felt unable to extricate herself from an unsatisfying affair with a married man. She managed to do that after two years of analysis. She is now a successful professional woman, managing a great deal of responsibility and authority, married, with two children. 'I love my husband, and I feel taken care of there. But I get something from you here that is different, and I need it.' She is hardly a candidate for a 'chronic ward,' yet there is something about her experience of dependency and need that remains part of our conversation, for now.

Surely, there are patients and therapists who become mired in long-term work, with little change or growth. Sometimes the sense of (mutual) dependence that can pervade such therapies reflects transference/countertransference impasses and enactments that may require interventions (consultations for therapist or patient) that can help to extricate the pair from treatments that have extended well past their proper 'expiration dates.' But I have far more often participated in analyses of long duration, as therapist, patient, and supervisor, in which new growth and healing continues to evolve and deepen as the years pass.

Sacks may have been correct in his estimation that his 50-year analysis with Shengold was testing the limits of how long an analysis might go, if only by virtue of the limits imposed by mortality itself. For an analytic couple to have a fifty-year relationship means that both have been blessed with long life.

Only very seasoned analysts and patients are in a position to speak from experience about the challenges of carrying on an analysis of decades-long duration. Freud observed in his late essay, 'Analysis Terminable and Interminable' (1937), that only very experienced analysts could speak from experience about whether a truly completed analysis is possible, since only such an analyst would be in a position to know about whether a patient he had seen could be said to be 'cured,' or whether further experience in life would suggest otherwise, as the patient returned to analysis later in life to take up problems left unaddressed the first time. To further complicate the question of when an analysis may be determined to be 'complete,' any given analyst's and patient's sense of what constitutes a completed analysis is relative to their sense of what analysis provides, what is possible, and when the analysis has gone far enough.

Till death do us part: is analysis a therapy without end?

It seemed that Sacks anticipated working with his therapist till death did them part. If he did remain in analysis until the end, he would not have been the first patient to come to the end of his life in analysis (Bass, 2001). Patients and analysts who work together for decades will sometimes eventually suffer the loss of one or the other, a loss that patients often imagine and anticipate. A supervisee recently told me about a session in which a patient, about to end her own therapy, asked her who would notify her 'if something happened.' A colleague whose analyst is now in his 90s told me today that he 'is waiting for that call—dreading it.' We make arrangements to notify our patients if we become ill or die, but not about former patients who are 'no longer with us.' Perhaps because of the unique structure of the therapeutic relationship, its frame and confidentiality, we have not developed the rituals for mourning that help in other kinds of personal relationships that eventually must come to an end. Woody Allen's joke (above) about the analyst continuing to charge for 'missed' sessions after death is perhaps carrying our tendency to deny the reality of death a bit far, even as it expresses the universal wish that important, intimate relationships could 'go on forever.'

Such wishes are not altogether unconflicted, of course. I have heard patients say, with some degree of guilt and embarrassment, that though they were sad that their analyst died, they also felt some degree of relief, as although they felt 'mostly ready to end therapy,' they hadn't seen a way that they could manage to 'really' end their therapy short of such extreme circumstances. Complicated responses such as these to 'forced' endings may reflect forms of ambivalence about dependency and separation that may be enacted and hidden for long periods of time in an analysis, and may become entangled with the analyst's own needs and blind spots. For example, when I asked a new patient whether she had spoken with her former analyst about her wish/fear of ending that analysis, which she told me had gone on for much longer than she felt was best for her, she indicated to me that it would have been impossible for her to do this—she would have hurt her the feelings of her analyst, whom she loved.

A final session

A patient recently 'finished' analysis after twenty years of therapy. After about a year of considering the prospect of coming to an end of our therapy, Jane was ready to set a date for our final session. We decided that it would be four months off, at our summer break.

During those four months, she continued to waver. Maybe she would change her mind. She would miss me, as I would miss her. What would it be like to experience the many difficult and important moments that life would inevitably bring, and that she had anticipated sharing with me, without having me to tell about them, she wondered? And what about my own death, which likely would come sooner than hers? Who would she talk to that about? There was her husband, of course, and friends. But telling **me** about the details of her emotional life in our twice/weekly sessions over the past twenty years had become an important part of that life.

She said, with tears in her eyes, that I had 'raised her,' and that leaving analysis felt like saying goodbye to a parent. She said she wanted to 'reserve the right' to come back. She believed she inevitably would. She was sure that there would be times in the future that she imagined that it would feel right to be talking again, whether for a short time (to tell me about the death of her parents, for example), or if something came up along the way that she felt would suggest further substantial work. 'I consider you my therapist for life, and as long as you are around, and in practice, I will think of you that way. I wouldn't want to see anyone else.'

In my experience, therapy ends in this way more often than not, with a patient considering the prospect of resuming therapy one day, even as s(he) reaches a sense that we have done enough for now. That may not be how 'terminating' analysis was traditionally conceived, at least theoretically, but why should it really be otherwise when therapy is regarded as a process of personal growth, healing and enrichment rather than promising an ultimate cure?

Analysis terminable in theory: interminable in practice?

Controversies about how long an analysis should take were present from the first days of analysis. Ferenczi (1955), in one of the first papers addressing the complexity of endings, highlighted the paradox of timelessness as a fundamental feature of the psychoanalytic situation, noting that the

> completion of an analysis is possible only if unlimited time is at one's disposal. By this I mean not so much the physical time at the patient's disposal, as his determination to persist for so long as may be necessary, irrespective of how long this may turn out to be.
>
> (p. 82)

In the same paper he suggested that 'a truly cured patient frees himself from analysis slowly but surely; he should continue to come to analysis as long as he wishes to' (p. 85). With one foot firmly planted in the classical perspective on transference, which he helped develop, even as he was disrupting it with new ideas about the analytic relationship, Ferenczi went on to say that

> the patient finally becomes convinced that he is continuing analysis only because he is treating it as a fantasy source of gratification, which in terms of reality, yields him nothing. When he has slowly overcome his mourning over this discovery, he inevitably looks around for other, more real sources of gratification. The renunciation of analysis is thus the final winding up of the infantile situation of frustration that lay at the basis of symptom formation.
>
> (1955, p. 85)

This perspective relies on a conception of analysis which holds that the analytic relationship is devoid of true gratifications and other meaningful rewards, so that once the patient is 'cured' of her neurosis, she will inevitably 'move on.'

Freud (1937) too struggled with the question of what is meant by the ambiguous term, 'the end of an analysis,' and how one might achieve it.

> An analysis is ended when analyst and patient cease to meet for the analytic session. This happens when two conditions have been approximately fulfilled. First, the patient must no longer be suffering from his former symptoms and must have overcome his various anxieties and inhibitions, and secondly, the analyst must have formed the opinion that so much repressed material has been brought into consciousness, so much that was inexplicable elucidated, and so much inner resistance overcome that no repetition of the patient's specific pathological process is to be feared.
>
> (p. 375)

'The second definition of the "end" is much more ambitious,' Freud (1937) continued.

> According to it we have to answer the question whether the effect upon the patient is so profound that we can be certain that no further change would take place in him if his analysis continued. The implication is that by means of analysis it is possible to attain to absolute psychic normality and be sure that it will be maintained, the supposition being that all the patient's repressions have been lifted and every gap in his memory filled.
>
> (p. 375)

The latter perspective relies on a conception of absolute normality, a goal in Freud's original conceptions that is not as convincing today. The question of when or whether an analysis is completed, which can be considered outside the subjective sphere of the two participants, is heavily reliant on theoretical considerations. 'We do not find it easy to answer these questions' (of analysis' ultimate terminability), without deferring to the 'magic of metapsychology' (1937, p. 381).

Freud's conclusion is that while one could imagine such an outcome in theoretical terms, in practical terms, analysis goes on. 'Every analyst ought periodically himself to submit to analysis, at intervals, of say, five years' (1937, p. 401). Similarly, in Ferenczi's last words on the matter, he noted the difference between what he believed to be possible and what he had in fact experienced in his daily practice of clinical psychoanalysis.

> I have brought all these observations to your notice today in support of my conviction that analysis is not an endless practice, but one which can be brought to a natural end with sufficient skill and patience on the analyst's part. If I am asked whether I can point to many such completed analyses, my answer must be 'no'.
>
> (1955, p. 86)

In these reflections we can see the awkward disjunction between theory and practice, when it comes to clarifying the question of just how far an analysis might go, beyond the experience of the two participants who must sort it out for themselves.

One patient's reflections on an unfinished (unfinishable?) analysis: not so crazy after all these (thirty-three) years

Sally first consulted me for therapy in 1985. We have spent approximately 5,000 hours speaking so far. We have talked about bringing our psychoanalytic conversations to a close several times over the years, but always find that there is more to talk about. We persist. Neither of us knows when or whether we will bring these conversations to a close. We have lived in Ferenczi's paradox, treating our time together as unlimited, even as we speak regularly about the passage of time and its finite nature. 'We have all the time in the world, even as we both recognize that our time is growing shorter.' She refers, from time to time, to such choice points, usually in the context of reflecting on the changes she has made since the last such juncture, and being glad that she has continued our conversation. She has talked recently about moving from New York, and raised the question in that context, of whether if she did move, I would consider continuing via Skype or phone. She is not ready to stop talking yet.

I recently told her that I was writing an essay (this chapter) on multi-decade-long analyses like ours, and that I would welcome her reflections on the matter. In the past few months, we have spent some time together, considering the long trajectory of our work so far, and she has been doing some reflective writing about her experience and recollections of the years we have spent together so far. In considering our long psychoanalytic collaboration, it seems apt to share some of her own reflections on the process.

When we met, I hadn't yet brought a case of analysis to completion, not even my own. I had worked with many patients who had 'stopped coming to therapy,' but I wouldn't have considered any of them a 'proper termination' of a therapeutic process, as I conceived that at the time. Thirty-five years into my practice, I have participated in thoughtfully planned endings to analyses many times. Each ending, like everything about analysis, is unique, unpredictable. No two analyses are alike; no two endings are alike. In each analysis, patient and analyst discover a pathway to the end of their work that is unlike any they have experienced before.

When Sally came to see me, she had reassured herself with an understanding that she had acquired in her reading, that analysis could be expected to last five to seven years, which seemed plausible enough to me at the time, though I already knew enough to know I didn't really know anything about how long she and I might meet. Notwithstanding her view that her analysis need not be a lifelong commitment, coming for help seemed risky. For one thing, getting help felt like a life or death matter, which she confirmed recently, looking back at a diary entry from early in our work. She wrote (in a journal that she recently shared with me) that she didn't think she could bear life in the absence of some significant change, even as such change felt out of reach. She hoped that psychoanalysis might make a difference, but she harbored significant doubts that this was possible, and if it wasn't, she felt her prospects for a future were dim. She has told me recently that something about her first few consultation sessions with me gave her a sense of hope, while she also experienced the dread of what would happen if things didn't work out with me (what if I decided that I could not work with her?).

On the other side of her concern that I would not take her into my practice was an equally compelling concern that she would never escape from it. She **must** not turn out to be like a cousin of hers, who had been in analysis all her adult life. The adults in Sally's family shook their heads in disdain at hapless Dotty's plight. She was the subject of many withering family discussions about the perils of interminable analysis. Sally's parents imagined and joked about the new wing of the therapist's house and the college educations that poor Dotty's problems had made possible for her fortunate psychiatrist.

Sally identified with Dotty.

> I remember how I experienced fear, terror really, of becoming like Dot. I knew I would be a pariah, which I guess I already was in my own mind at least. It was the state that I was in then. It wasn't a good state.

And it wasn't truly my own mind, which I was to some extent 'out of.' It was the mindset of my family. It was too shameful for me to realize I was like Dotty. My mind was split between my (secret) identification with her and my betrayal of her. I couldn't own that identification so I withdrew from her. I realize in saying her name now, feeling it come off my tongue, that 'Dotty' also stood for 'crazy' … It seemed like a term of endearment in a way, but there was nothing truly endearing about it. It was always said with some degree of disdain. I was confused by it. I loved Dotty at the same time that I shared my parent's pity for her, and feared that I was her. We never called her Dorothy, which was actually her name.

I remember feeling, when we started, 'please don't let me, whatever happens, turn into Dot.' She was always measured by what she would have been or could have been, but shamefully, mortifyingly, was not. Dot would arrive at the house and sometimes be put together, in respect to her attire and appearance, but most often, she would be askew or akimbo somehow with a falling hem or a sweater oddly buttoned, lipstick applied like a wobbly gash. Her gait was awkward. Her weight fluctuated. Sound familiar? I am describing myself. There were positive identifications too, mainly secret. I remember her as curiously warm, and interesting and interested in me. She may have been the only person in my family who I felt was interested in me. People in the family air-kissed her, in a dismissive way. They kept a distance between her body and theirs. I maintained that distance with my weight. No one could get too close to my body, the fat was in between. I kept in control of the distance. But I did embrace Dot and she embraced me. There must have been a part of me that knew she was the realest person in the family, but another part that realized that to see her clearly (she was smart, a writer, empathic) meant to deny and defy the family. I was forced to make a choice. I was obligated to fade her away, scorn her, to see crazy Dotty, not loving and creative Dorothy. Or I would face a similar fate. I did suffer her fate, while trying to avoid it. You are your relationships. You can't choose your family. Yet in a sense one does later. I have chosen to stay in analysis with you. I feel that there is something about all these years with you—they begin to add up, and to make things possible that wouldn't have been possible without them.

I have a keen sense memory of rejecting Dorothy, of her becoming Dot to me, and the betrayal of her, and so of myself, that flowed like acid in me. I remember the hardening of my heart against her, the anger toward her, the closing of my mind against her. I know you have seen me close my mind and harden my heart. It is, or has been, one of my deepest shames. One of my several big regrets. I didn't know until recently that I was hardening my heart against myself too, against the

> Dotty in me. Reclaiming parts of myself that I didn't even know were there or missing has been an important part of what our work has made possible
>
> I remember in my first sessions, telling you with such forcefulness how I definitely did not want to end up like Dot. I did not want to be in analysis forever, though I am now sure that a part of me must have wanted that. I was secretly relieved when you made no promises about that. When I said I figured that analysis might be five to seven years, you didn't disagree. But when I asked what you thought, you said it would depend on what we found along the way, and for how long I would find it useful. It has not been forever, but close to it. And I am still finding it more than useful. Part of what has happened here is that I have reclaimed the Dorothy in me, while making the Dot in me less shameful and dreadful.
>
> As I have come to see more Dorothy in Dotty I am both more and less 'Dotty.' A long drawn out treatment was terrifying, the kiss of death. But then so was intimacy. It wasn't just the kiss of death I was avoiding, but the kiss of life. That was beyond me then but starting to be reclaimed now because of the many iterations of shame and despair that we have gone through here, before I could reclaim something on the other side of that.
>
> I remember at the start of therapy with you, Jenny called me frigid, and your typically unanxious reframe of that. You asked with your gentle curiosity if I felt 'frozen,' which allowed for something other than shame—an accepting curiosity that was like the seed of something that has taken root over all these years. Being frigid was not a death sentence, or a humiliation, but maybe a way of beginning to think about how things got frozen in the first place. I began to feel a growing capacity to rely upon and trust you, to register my dissociative states as a start to finding out more. I know that we could not have arrived at this point, the work we have done in the last few sessions, with new life for me seeming possible even as my parents are finally coming to the end of theirs.

Sally recently said about a difficult conversation we had, that here is no way that she could have had this conversation ten years ago, even ten weeks ago or last week.

> I feel that what we are talking about now would have been too hard to bear; how we went today from your noticing that I was making a kind of speech that you couldn't quite follow, to making the kind of contact that we are making now. It makes me realize more about where I was when I came in, and where I am now in making contact with myself and with you.

Analysis has become an enriching part of Sally's life, with ongoing benefits that go far beyond any original expectations that either of us could have anticipated of what analysis might bring because those expectations were generated before the therapeutic relationship made other ways of being and relating possible.

Over time, the therapeutic relationship that we developed made it possible for Sally to feel recognized in and to recognize all of the disparate parts of herself: the Dotty, the Dorothy, and all the rest. Gradually she began to recognize that the 'Dotty' part that came to sessions askew and akimbo, and the parts of herself that were warm, generous, smart and talented were part of the whole person that she was increasingly becoming and coming to like. We found that the relationship we developed in our many years in analysis made it possible for her to gradually surrender the need to protectively keep these parts of herself separated as her sense of herself became more and more whole over time. Notwithstanding her original view that a long analysis would exacerbate the very shame that she hoped to ease, her experience in analysis made possible a different kind of relationship with me and with herself than could have been imagined when we started.

Making a decision to end our relationship would be a far more complicated challenge than we could have anticipated the day we met, analyst/patient/strangers. As in many analyses, the patient has become capable, through the analytic work, of a far richer experience than was possible before the analysis. In ending our work, far from Ferenczi's (1955) belief that we will recognize that we are giving up less than we thought, we will find that we are giving up something that we have discovered with each other along the way, which could not possibly have been anticipated when we began.

End points and new beginnings

Each analytic journey is unique, entirely unpredictable as to the time any given patient and therapist will spend together. Most analytic patients and their analysts eventually recognize that they have carried their work as far as they can, or as far as they are prepared to go at that time. The realization of an end point in a fruitful analysis often takes many years to accomplish and even after a decade or two or more of intense analytic work, endings may remain elusive, with patients feeling that the benefits of continuing analysis outweigh the costs.

Endings remain uncertain. Each analytic couple forges a path that inevitably traverses unexpected terrain. Analyst and patient alike change along the way, opening new paths of exploration that could not have been anticipated. Each patient's (and analyst's) sense of what might be a desirable and achievable goal of analysis over time will inevitably change along the way, as awareness expands, perspectives shift, and the patient comes to see emergent aspects of what brought her to analysis in the first place, and what might constitute an acceptable end point. Each patient's response to the question 'what brings you here?' will be quite different in the first session from what it will be five years later, or ten or twenty. With patients like Sally, and others I have seen for many years, that ultimately remains to be seen.

References

Balint, M. (1950). On the termination of analysis. *Int. J. Psycho-Anal.*, *31*, 196–199.

Bass, A. (2001). It takes one to know one: Or, whose unconscious is it anyway? *Psychoanal. Dialogues*, *11*(5), 683–702.

Ferenczi, S. (1955). *The problem of the termination of the analysis in final contributions to the problems and methods of psychoanalysis.* New York: Brunner/Mazel.

Freud, S. (1953). Jokes and their relation to the unconscious. In *The standard edition of the complete psychological works of Sigmund Freud*, Volume VIII (pp. 1–247). London: Hogarth Press.

Freud, S. (1937). Analysis terminable and interminable. *Int. J. Psycho-Anal.*, *18*, 373–405.

Sacks, O. (2011). 'The longest running psychoanalysis on record.' Retrieved from www.webofstories.com/play/oliver.sacks/196.

Index

abandonment 69, 79, 154
Abrams, Jane 152–165
abuse 12, 30, 41, 46, 52, 110, 119; bearing witness 8; by father 44, 45, 76, 77–78, 79, 81; helplessness of therapist 123, 124; memories of 112, 135; by mother 119, 136; by neighbor 121; partner 63
action plans 158–159, 160, 161–162
adaptational strength 40
addiction 11
affect regulation 33, 80
affective neuroscience 158
agency 11, 25, 115, 156
Ainsworth, Mary 102
alcohol abuse 40, 41
alienation 10
Allen, Woody 7, 166, 169–170, 174
alpha function 101, 103, 104, 111, 112, 115
Alvarez, Anne 103–104
ambivalence 64, 147, 148, 172, 174
ambivalent attachment 102
American Psychoanalytic Association 171
anger 18–19, 21, 76, 79, 80; emotional convictions 11; response to dreams 113–114; terminally ill patients 133; therapists 126; unconscious 112; *see also* rage
Annie Hall 166
anxiety 9, 24, 28–29, 43, 154; disorganized attachment 79; emotional convictions 11; therapist's 135
Arendt, Hannah 124
Arlow, Jacob 3, 6
Aron, L. 66
art 16, 21–22
Asperger's syndrome 17
assessment 10, 25
attachment 13, 99, 101, 102; avoidant 102, 104, 106; disorganized 79–80, 97, 102; dysfunctional patterns 35; insecure 102, 103, 109; mentalization 102–103; safety 154; secure 97, 102, 103, 114; trauma 153, 161–162, 163
attachment theory 31–32
attunement 89, 162
Atwood, G. 15, 18
autism 17
"auto-biology" 160
autonomy 82, 83, 104, 145
avoidant attachment 102, 104, 106

Back, A. L. 124
"bad objects" 69, 145, 156, 167
Baer, D. 125
Bass, Anthony 145, 146, 166–182
bearing witness 8, 122, 136–137, 163
Beebe, B. 75
Benjamin, J. 153, 155, 156, 157
bereavement 30, 31, 61–63, 125–126; death of a son 149, 150; suffering 122; therapist's experience of 68, 135; *see also* death; loss; mourning
Bergmann, Martin S. 3, 54, 133, 142
Berzoff, Joan 119–131, 134
beta elements 103
Bettleheim, Bruno 38
biology 160–161
Bion, Wilfred 98, 101, 103, 104, 111, 122
Blanck, Gertrude and Ruben 3, 6
Bloom, Victor 53–54
Blum, L. 125
Bollas, C. 144
boundary invasion 147
Bowlby, John 101, 102

brain development 33
brief treatment 6, 9, 10, 13, 37–41, 51
Bromberg, Philip 91, 92, 136
Browning, David 125–126
Broyard, Anatole 123, 124
Buddhism 17, 122
bullying 29, 52
burnout 126
Byock, I. 133–134

Calhoun, L. G. 122
cancer 123, 132–133, 135–136, 139–140
Care System 158
change 47, 122–123, 159–160, 162
chemotherapy 136, 139–140
children: attachment theory 102; child development 33; disorganized attachment 79–80; *Infant Care* bulletin 37
Chinese culture 75, 76–77, 78, 83
Christianity 122
closeness 34, 66, 68, 69, 154, 162; *see also* intimacy
communication 4
compassion 81–82, 87, 119, 124–125, 134
compassion fatigue 126
complementarity 155, 157
confidentiality 4
Confucian worldview 76–77
connection 24, 25
container/contained 98, 101, 104, 111, 115
containment 92, 104, 115
conversation 20
costs 9–10, 25
countertransference 34, 74, 78–79, 156; enactments 66, 173; group supervision 127; negative impact of 8; sadomasochism 89; unbearable 99
couple's work 105, 109–110
criticism 154–155, 156
crying 108, 139, 149
culture 75, 76–77, 79, 83, 158
Currow, D. C. 123

DasGupta, S. 124
Davies, Jody Messler 65, 69, 70, 71, 98, 153–154
death: of analyst 6, 132, 135–136, 174; of client 133–134, 137, 139–140, 171, 174; of sibling 80; *see also* bereavement
defenses 40, 101, 107, 109, 114, 157, 158–159
deficit, theory of 104
delusions 15–16
denial 40, 79
dependency 7, 34, 143, 173, 174
depression 30, 43, 44, 50, 150; "auto-biology" 160; emotional convictions 11; managed care 39; postpartum 91; therapists 126
deprivation 7, 46, 154
developmental perspective 33–34, 35, 101
DeYoung, Patricia 9–26
diagnosis 10
Diagnostic and Statistical Manual of Mental Disorders (DSM-V) 11
differentiation 82
disorganized attachment 79–80, 97, 102
dissociation 80, 97, 104, 110, 114; emotional convictions 11; enactments 157; psychosis 115; as response to trauma 92; right-brain regulation 20; splitting 13
distress 11, 24, 25, 103
Doidge, N. 28
Dragosei, Angela Connolly 27
dreams 64, 67, 111–112, 113–114, 166; inability to distinguish hallucinations from 103, 104; repressed memories 152; therapist's 91, 92, 93, 97; *see also* nightmares
DSM-V *see* Diagnostic and Statistical Manual of Mental Disorders
dysregulation 21, 24, 30, 32

eating disorders 41
Edward, Joyce 3–8
Edwards, N. 134
Egnew, T. R. 122
ego 122, 158
ego strength 39–40, 114
Eichmann, Adolf 124
emotional development 33
emotional pain 10, 11
emotions 76, 78, 108; attachment theory 102; barriers to expression of 107; homeostatic affects 158; toleration of 109
empathy 81–82, 115, 121, 124, 134, 150, 158
enactments 61, 65–66, 153–154, 162; repetition 157; self-loss 15;

silences 64; transference 13, 173; uncertainty 159
enmeshment 154
ethics 8, 34
exploitation 35

failed witness 155, 156–157
Fairbairn, W. R. D. 152, 153, 161, 163
Fargione, Kathleen 101–116
fear 81, 108, 154; acceptance of 76, 82; disorganized attachment 79, 80; Fear System 158; hiding 83; unconscious 112
Ferenczi, S. 175–176, 177, 181
Figley, C. R. 126
flashbacks 44, 45, 80
Fonagy, Peter 102–103
Fox, Richard 94
fragmentation 13, 14, 15, 24, 69, 114
Frank, Arthur 121
Frankl, Viktor 122–123
Freud, Sigmund 121, 122, 160, 169, 173, 176–177
Friedman, Lawrence 3
friendship 143
Frosh, S. 62
funding 39

Galassi, S. 99
Ganzer, Carol 61–73
Gaudilliere, Jean-Max 70
gender roles 76
"ghosts" 62, 70–71, 122
Glennon, Stefanie Solow 141–151
good-enough care 41–42, 46, 99
"good objects" 61, 65, 68, 69–70, 115, 153, 167
Good, P. R. 37
gratitude 92, 99, 133
grief 30, 31, 71, 76, 80; loss of mother 95, 97; Panic/Grief System 158; shared experience of 149, 150; suffering 121, 122, 126; terminal illness 137; *see also* loss; mourning
group supervision 126–127
guilt 45, 80, 81; about long-term work 172; failed witness 156; homeostatic affects 158; terminal illness 132, 133; unresolved 97
Guntrip, H. 152–153, 154, 161, 163, 164

Halifax, J. S. 124, 126
hallucinations 15, 103, 104, 112, 115
Halpert, E. 39
Harris, Adrienne 65, 69
healing 71, 98, 104, 115, 162, 164, 175
health insurance 39, 47, 50–51
Hegarty, M. 123
helplessness 80, 81–82, 119, 155; suffering 120, 121, 123–124; therapist's 86, 123–124, 132, 156
Hitchcock, Robyn 94
HIV 28–29
holding 42, 119, 133, 159–160
holding environment 41–42, 48, 154, 162–163
Holocaust 122, 129
homeostatic affects 158
homosexuality 29, 52
hospitalization 45, 46, 50–51, 54–55
hostility 11, 23
humiliation 77–78
hypervigilance 11, 137

identity 75
illness 6–7; terminal 119, 132–140
imagination 124
immigrants 75–76, 77, 82
impasses 61, 67, 69, 71, 83, 153; mourning 65, 70; mutual recognition 155; transference/countertransference 173; uncertainty 159
impulse control 40
individuation 145
Infant Care bulletin (1914) 37
insecure attachment 102, 103, 109
insurance plans 39, 47, 50–51
integration 113–114, 115
interminability 141–146, 173–174, 175–177
internal objects 65, 67–68, 101, 114, 145, 167; *see also* "bad objects"; "good objects"; object relations
intersubjectivity 12, 31–32, 65, 152, 157, 159
intimacy 141, 149–150, 151, 162–163; autonomy valued over 104; fear of 180; study on therapists' experiences 34; terminal illness 137
introjection 103, 115
intrusion 147
invalidation 15, 16
isolation 9, 10, 24

jokes 166, 169
joy 115, 128–129
Judaism 121–122
Jungian therapy 31–32

Kahn, M. W. 55
Kalb, M. 70
Kanter, J. 42
Kaszniak, A. W. 124
Klein, Melanie 99
Kohut, H. 89
Kotcher, Jean 27–36
Kramer, P. D. 47
Kubler-Ross, E. 134

learning 158; from experience 122
Lee, Arthur 94
Levenson, Ed 144
Levinas, E. 121, 124
Levine, Peter 104
Loewald, Hans 33–34, 122
long-distance therapy 52
long-term treatment 9–10, 13; assumptions 11, 12, 25; characteristics of long-term patients 32–33; clinical value of 35; criticism of 27, 35; Edward on 4–6, 7–8; growing old together 171–172; interminability 141–146, 173–174, 175–177; patient's reflections on 177–181; Sacks 53, 170–171, 173, 174; study on therapists' experiences 27–28, 31–32, 34; trauma 61, 72; unconventional 74–75
Lord, Susan 3–8, 132–140, 141, 142, 145, 163
Lorenz, Konrad 102
loss 61, 63, 119, 128; characteristics of long-term patients 32, 35; internalization of lost object 122; of mother 95, 97; terminal illness 137; therapist's own experience of 125, 127; unmourned 71; *see also* bereavement; grief; mourning
love 54, 94, 99, 133, 150
Lust System 158

MacDuffie, K. 160
Mackenzie, K. R. 40–41
Mahler, Margaret 3
managed care 3–4, 39, 43, 47, 50–51
management 42
Marino, Gordon 75
maternal reverie 98
Mayer, E. 134
McGleughlin, J. 69, 70, 71
McWilliams, Nancy 96
meaninglessness 123
medication 11, 14, 15, 25, 53; antidepressant 43, 150; cost of 9; symptom relief 10
melancholia 122
melancholy object 62, 72
memory/memories 160, 164; of abuse 112, 135; disorganized attachment 79; inability to distinguish dreams from 103, 104; neuropsychoanalysis 153, 158, 159, 161; repressed 152
mental disorders 10, 11
mentalization 102–103
Meyer, William S. 37–49, 50–58
miscarriage 96–97, 106, 110, 172
Mitchell, S. A. 66
Modell, A. 41
mortality 123
mother-infant relationship 41, 46
motivation 40, 74
mourning 31, 61–62, 63, 135; end of therapeutic relationship 174; incomplete 150; suffering 122, 126; therapeutic impasses 65, 70, 71; unresolved 61, 67, 70, 72
music 19, 20, 21, 88, 93–94, 138
mutual recognition 75, 155
mutual regulation 19–20

narcissism: therapist's 66–67; traumatic 77–78
needs 158, 161
neglect 12, 32, 35, 46, 62, 69
Neimeyer, R. A. 122
neuropsychoanalysis 153, 154, 157–159, 161
night terrors 45, 88, 138–139
nightmares 43, 45, 80, 110, 111–112, 113, 115
"normalcy" 10, 114
Nouwen, Henri 121, 125, 128–129

object relations 31–32, 65, 70, 89, 101, 103–104; *see also* "bad objects"; "good objects"; internal objects
objectification 10, 15, 16, 21
Ogden, Pat 104, 109

Ogden, T. H. 98
Osbon, A. 99

pain 79, 81, 89, 121; emotional 10, 11; helplessness of therapist 124; sharing 125, 128
Panic/Grief System 158
Panksepp, Jaak 158
parallel process 47
parents 29, 30, 83, 107; disorganized attachment 79–80; dreams about 112; *Infant Care* bulletin 37; mentalization 102–103; parent-child relationship 33–34, 41, 46
Patchen, Kenneth 127
Peacock-Corral, Natalie 86–100
Perry, Bruce 104, 111
Play System 158
Poland, Warren 27, 35
pregnancy 90, 92, 93, 96–97
prevention 12
primary processes 112, 158
privacy 4
productivity 10
projection 40, 67, 70, 89, 99, 153–154, 157
projective identification 89, 124, 153–154, 157
psychic development 101, 110
psychic structure 101, 107, 109, 114
psychodynamic therapy 153
psychological mindedness 40, 86
psychosis 14, 15, 115

racism 119, 120, 121, 123
rage 18–19, 45, 86, 88, 95–96, 114; father's 77; internalized 81; Rage System 158; surviving a patient's 92; terminally ill patients 132, 133; therapist's 156; *see also* anger
rape 44, 64, 110, 112; *see also* sexual abuse
Rattner, M. 123
recognition 67, 75, 155, 157
Redding, K. K. 134
regression 95, 135
regulation 19–20; *see also* self-regulation
relational instability 11
relational psychoanalysis 9–10, 12, 92–93; interminability 141, 142, 145–146; non-pathologizing 14; short-term 13; study on long-term treatment 31–32
relationships 30–31, 62, 63, 67, 81–82, 114; *see also* therapeutic relationship
religion 17, 121–122
repetition compulsion 157, 160
repression 153, 154, 157–158, 159, 160, 164
resilience 13, 128
retirement 7
reverie 87, 98
Rezenbrink, I. 125, 127
right-brain regulation 19–20
Ringel, Shoshana 74–85
Roland, A. 76–77
Rushton, C. H. 124
Russell, P. 156, 161, 162, 164

Sacks, Oliver 52–53, 170–171, 173, 174
sadness 7, 76, 77, 80, 81
sadomasochistic object relations 89, 93
safety 102, 104, 115, 150, 154, 163
Schaefer, R. 89
Schafer, Roy 3
schizophrenia 14, 17
Schore, A. 19–20
Searles, Harold 92
The Secret Garden 94
secure attachment 97, 102, 103, 114
Seeking System 158
self: bicultural 83; Confucian concept of 76–77; core sense of 19; experiences of 11; fragmented 13, 14, 15, 114; suffering 121
self-awareness 13
self-blame 79, 156
self-care 88, 89
self-concept 21
self-destruction 96
self-determination 4
self-disclosure 68–69
self-esteem 21, 32, 44
self-harm 11, 30, 88, 114, 135, 138
self-hatred 81
self-knowledge 162, 164
self-loathing 9, 10, 18, 45
self-loss 15
self-organization 33, 76
self-reflection 11, 25, 92
self-regulation 19, 20, 21, 33
self-reliance 82, 83
self-states 65, 66, 69–70, 79, 80–81, 92, 155, 156
self-supervision 8

Semrad, Elvin 38
"sentinel effect" 47, 51
separation 145, 158, 174
sex addiction 88
sexual abuse 41, 110; by father 44, 45; helplessness of therapist 124; memories of 112, 135; by mother 136; by neighbor 121; *see also* abuse
sexuality 29
shame 77–78, 81, 167, 180, 181; acceptance of 76; disorganized attachment 79, 80; homeostatic affects 158; overcoming 83; terminal illness 133; therapist's 34, 145, 155, 156, 157, 172–173
Shaw, D. 77
Shedler, J. 153
Shengold, Leonard 53, 170–171, 173
silences 30, 64, 66
Silverman, P. R. 134
Slade, A. 102
Slavin, M. 134
Sleeper 169–170
Solms, Mark 157, 158–159
splitting 13, 157
stability 5, 34
Stolorow, Robert 125
Stone, L. 40
Strauman, T. 160
stress 12, 21
subjective being 10, 25
substance abuse 40, 41, 52–53, 86, 98, 170
suffering 10, 119–128, 154, 161
suicidality 7, 11, 30, 40, 51–52, 95, 110, 120
superego 122
superiority 11
supervision 89, 126–127
"supportive psychotherapy" 55
Symington, J. and N. 111, 112

Tedeschi, R. G. 122
terminal illness 119, 132–140
termination 135, 143–144, 174–175, 181–182; contacting former patients 147; Ferenczi 175–176; Freud 176–177; human relationships 133; patient's comments on 141–142, 148; patient's desire for 125–126; planned endings 178; premature 40; pressure for 53; study on therapists' experiences 32; therapist's lack of experience of 172–173; *see also* interminability
therapeutic relationship 5, 35, 61, 133, 163, 181; action plans 161; end of 174; healing 98; holding environment 41–42, 154; impact of managed care 4; interminability 141, 142; internalization of the 145; as love relationship 54; modes of working 11; mother-infant relationship comparison 41; mutuality 172; study on therapists' experiences 34; toleration of uncertainty 159
therapists: death of 6, 132, 135–136, 174; enactments 65–66; good-enough 41–42; study on long-term treatment 27–28, 31–32, 34
third-party reimbursement 39, 47
time-limited treatment 6
timelessness 175
Toffler, Alvin 38, 47
transference 19, 74, 78–79, 168; enactments 13, 66, 173; Ferenczi 175–176; Guntrip 163; idealizing 91; maternal 152; positive 63, 75
transformation 122–123
trauma 9, 61–73, 74, 86; attachment trauma 153, 161–162, 163; characteristics of long-term patients 32, 35; containment 115; developmental 99; disorganized attachment 79–80, 102; impact on human development 7; neuropsychoanalysis 154; relational 11, 104; repressed memory of 152; trauma theory 20–21, 104; traumatic narcissism 77–78; working through 80–82; *see also* abuse
Tresan, David 27, 31, 35
Tronick, E. Z. 162
trust 35, 61, 105, 109; building 107, 108; developmental perspective 33; homeostatic affects 158; integration 114; sacred 163; therapeutic relationship 133; toleration of uncertainty 159, 160

uncertainty 32, 159–160

validation 15, 16, 67, 76, 78
van der Kolk, Bessel 104

volatility 11
vulnerability 12, 16, 21, 78–79, 81, 107; acceptance of 76; hiding 80, 83; self-loss 15

Wallerstein, Robert 32
well-being 10, 11, 24
Wiesel-Barth, J. 74–75
window of tolerance 109, 114
Winnicott, Donald W. 41–42, 46, 92, 98, 152–153, 161
women 80, 120–121
"wounded healer" 121
"wounding healer" 155

yoga 22–23, 24

Zuckerman, R. L. 39

For Product Safety Concerns and Information please contact our EU representative GPSR@taylorandfrancis.com
Taylor & Francis Verlag GmbH, Kaufingerstraße 24, 80331 München, Germany

www.ingramcontent.com/pod-product-compliance
Ingram Content Group UK Ltd.
Pitfield, Milton Keynes, MK11 3LW, UK
UKHW020203200926
475702UK00004B/586
* 9 7 8 0 3 6 7 1 5 0 1 5 0 *